WISDOM FROM THOSE IN CARE

ALSO BY CONNIE GOLDMAN

Tending the Earth, Mending the Spirit:
The Healing Gifts of Gardening (with Richard Mahler)

The Ageless Spirit: Reflections on Living Life to the Fullest in Midlife and the Years Beyond

The Gifts of Caregiving: Stories of Hardship, Hope, and Healing, Second Edition

Late Life Love: Romance and New Relationships in Later Years

Secrets of Becoming a Late Bloomer: Staying Creative, Aware, and Involved in Midlife and Beyond (with Richard Mahler)

Who Am I . . . Now That I'm Not Who I Was:
Conversations with Women in Midlife and Beyond

've
WISDOM FROM
THOSE IN CARE

CONVERSATIONS, INSIGHTS, AND INSPIRATION

Connie Goldman

THE PARTNERS IN CAREGIVING PROJECT

WISDOM FROM THOSE IN CARE ©2018 by Connie Goldman. All rights reserved. No part of this publication may be used or reproduced in any manner whatsoever without written permission, except in the case of brief quotations embodied in critical articles and reviews. For further information, please contact the publisher.

THE SOCIETY OF CERTIFIED SENIOR ADVISORS

The Society of Certified Senior Advisors (SCSA) is the leading certifying organization for multidisciplinary professionals who have prepared themselves to work more effectively with older adults through education, training, continuing education and a professional code of eithcs.

Professionals who hold the competency-based CSA® designation have distinguished themselves by demonstrating knowledge and understanding of the multiple processes of aging that affect the biological, behavioral, social, and economic aspects of the life course. The CSA® certification is accredited by both the National Commission for Certifying Agencies (NCCA) and the American National Standards Institute (ANSI) meeting the highest standards of quality assurance available in personnel certification.

SCSA promotes knowledge exchange in the field of aging through traditional and new media channels including its award winning *Working With Older Adults* curriculum, the *CSA Journal,* educational webinars, conferences, workshops, newsletters, social media and local leadership groups.

Library of Congress Control Number: 2018931874
ISBN: 978-0-9762451-2-4
Design: Stylus Creative
Printing: CEC Document Services Press

To all who are now or have been in family care. Something in each of your stories nourishes both courage and acceptance.

CONTENTS

VIII	Foreword
X	Preface
XI	Acknowledgments
1	Introduction
7	Tasha – I Came to Believe I Could
15	David – Acceptance and Contentment
25	Julie – He's with Me for the Journey
35	Dianne – Enjoying My Life
43	Betty – I Found a New Life
49	Carol – This Isn't Going to Spoil My Day
55	Bob – I Can Still Sing and Laugh
63	Suleika – I'm a Winner
71	Marge – Positive Ways to Live
77	Rona – My Sensible and Life-Affirming View
81	Kenneth – Continued Learning and Comfort
89	Susie – Surrounded by Love
99	Susan – An Attitude of Regeneration
105	Barry – Winning My Battle
115	Lasha – Life's Slow Recovery
123	Jeff – Living Each Day Fully
135	Suz – Life in a Support Community
141	Sandra – Finding Optimism and Peace
147	Marcus – A New Normal
155	Ken – Life's Many Good Days
165	Ruth – Life Is Full of Joy
173	Katrina – A Good Life
181	Gary – A Life of Helping Others
189	Bill – Helping Others Seek a Good Life
195	Ron – I Live in the Ever-Present Present
203	Afterword

FOREWORD

IT'S HARD TO BELIEVE THERE WAS A TIME WHEN STORIES ABOUT growing older were rare in the media. Most people hope to live a long life, and perhaps we would rather not think about what can happen if we become injured, frail, or, even worse, "demented." People with such challenges are generally absent from television, radio, and other media sources; producers may fear the images and voices of those who don't fit the "norm" will not attract audiences.

Yet in the early 1980s, Connie Goldman boldly set out to share on public radio stories about many facets of growing older, focusing on the lives of well-known people and those who live so-called ordinary lives. Even those without name recognition offered their gifts, and in her renowned book about caregivers, entitled *The Gifts of Caregiving: Stories of Hardship, Hope, and Healing,* Goldman crafted the experiences of people who care for others using their own words, showering us with inspiration and offering seeds of contemplation.

This companion book, *Wisdom from Those in Care: Conversations, Insights, and Inspiration,* focuses on persons receiving care and illustrates that caregiving and being cared for are intertwined. People in need of care still care about others, and their own gifts of spirit, determination, resilience, and realism flow through their stories—in their own words. No other book has so richly revealed the reflections of people who have navigated the terrain of illness or disability, learning how to accept help and ultimately partner with helpers to grow together.

In the lives of the people whose rich stories unfold in *Wisdom from Those in Care,* Goldman opens a window that goes beyond the stated words of conversations. A philosophy of living, a crucible moment of insight, and an appreciation of the experience of being *in need of care* emerge. We are given an opportunity to identify with the person who needs a wheelchair or whose head is bald from the side effects of chemotherapy, or even experiences a silent disability that is revealed through a pained expression of someone whose every move reflects a deeper physical or emotional pain.

In this book of thoughts—the thoughts of those who have received care and of Goldman, and the thoughts she encourages you to consider—we are offered the pot of gold at *each* end of the rainbow. It shows us that offering and receiving care are on a spectrum. And as Ram Dass notes in *Polishing the Mirror: How to Live from Your Spiritual Heart,* we are all souls, not our roles. This soulful expression of survival, resilience, and passion for living in the collective stories shared by Connie Goldman is a welcome gift.

Read on and reflect, share, and, most of all, care.

Connie Corley, MSW, MA, PhD
Professor, Fielding Graduate University
January 16, 2017

PREFACE

THIS BOOK HAD A LONG PREGNANCY. IT IS A COMPANION TO MY book of stories told by family caregivers, *The Gifts of Caregiving: Stories of Hardship, Hope, and Healing.* Those caregivers speak of their many responsibilities, stress, and exhaustion, and their new learning about themselves resulting from their caregiver commitments. One day I was visiting a friend now receiving home-based care who was dealing with advanced cancer. Her daughter had moved into my friend's home and become full-time caregiver for her mother. I told her daughter to take the afternoon off and that I would stay with and care for her mother's needs.

Her mother and I had been friends for many years, and I had become a more frequent visitor as her mother's condition was quickly declining. That afternoon we shared a conversation of considerable depth. My friend looked back on her family relations and her work and travel experiences in her long life. She shared far more than facts, revealing deep feelings that I had never heard her express before. I suspected that much of what she talked about might not have been shared with anyone previously. My role that day was just to be a listener. That experience gave me a new perspective: the person in care could have a different point of view and understanding of the caregiving experience.

I've shared the stories I've collected over many years in programs I've produced for pubic radio, offered speeches and workshops at conferences, and written many articles and a half dozen books. The stories I've shared are the words of those who have told me their personal experiences. My wish is that the stories you'll read in this book will bring you, or someone you know, both information and inspiration. I sincerely believe that sharing a personal story can offer an unexpected gift of both hope and healing.

ACKNOWLEDGMENTS

I OFFER MANY THANKS TO ALL THE PEOPLE RECEIVING CARE who have shared with me their personal stories and experiences. Please accept my gratitude, too, for granting the permission to share your stories in this book. Each person was open and honest about changes in physical health and the ways he or she learned to accept care from others. Those in care talked of the challenges of adapting to new limitations and often difficult adjustments. My appreciation and thanks to all who helped make this book a reality.

Many thanks and a bundle of gratitude to Kay Whaley, my friend and my efficient office helper. Also appreciation and thanks to my editor and dear friend, Beth Gaede, who has been here for me through ups and downs. She has been the midwife to the birth of this book and many of my other writings.

My endless thanks to my daughter, Nancy Goldman, and my son, Barry Goldman, for encouraging me during the long pregnancy of this book, and to friends and colleagues who encouraged me with words like "Stick with it," "This book says something important," and "No one else has written a book about the people receiving care."

I'm especially grateful for the encouragement and help of my now deceased, late-life partner, Ken Tilsen. Without his encouragement, and a couple of laughs a day, you might not have had this book in your hands.

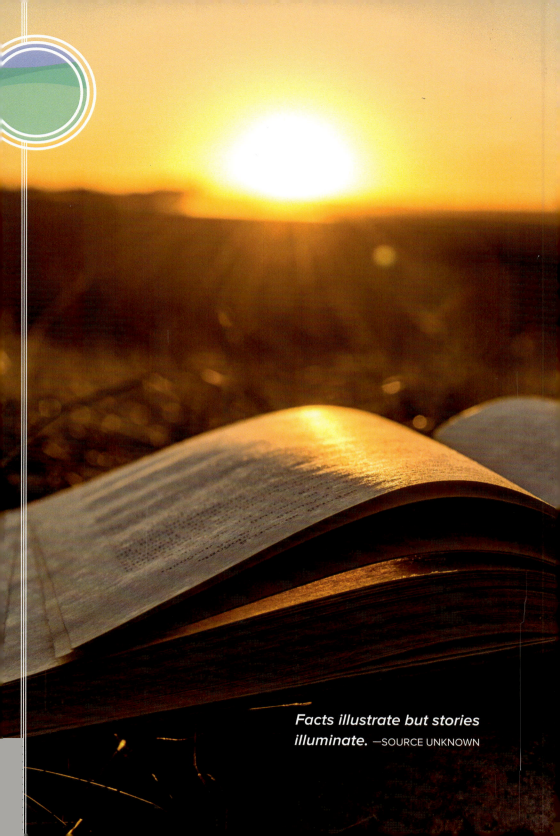

Facts illustrate but stories illuminate. —SOURCE UNKNOWN

INTRODUCTION

SO HERE ARE THE FACTS. SURVEY FINDINGS DIFFER, BUT A 2015 report released by the Family Caregiver Alliance indicated there were at that time 43.5 million family caregivers in America. No doubt that figure has increased since then, but both then and now, it represents enormous diversity in the ages of those receiving family care and the reasons they need help.

I could provide many more facts about family caregiving, but like many other people, I believe in the power of stories to communicate important ideas. Through my years as a public radio reporter, author, and speaker, I have seen stories illuminate in a way that "Just the facts, Ma'am" cannot. Because stories communicate so effectively, several of the books I have written are composed primarily of peoples' stories, framed by insights I have drawn from them.

In my book *The Gifts of Caregiving: Stories of Hardship, Hope, and Healing,* I offer conversations with family caregivers. They generously shared with me their personal learning and insights and described changes in their lives during or after their time as a primary family caregiver. Each caregiver I spoke with talked about the needs of the person in their care. They shared stories of frustration, stress, uncertainty, and guilt as drastic alterations in their family life and jobs made their days as a caregiver more demanding. Yet they reported that along with the hardships and losses, their caregiver experience often offered a gift in disguise—an experience that resulted in more meaningful and deeper connections with the person they cared for and also with themselves.

One conversation I had with a caregiver, which I related at length in *The Gifts of Caregiving,* brought to my attention how rewarding listening to and hearing the voice of the person in care can be. The caregiver was an adult son taking care of his father. Here is some of his story as I recall it:

> I would get done working at the college, see my private clients, get to my dad's house at seven at night, make his dinner, change his bed, do the laundry, give him his medication, clean the house, get his meals ready for the next day, and leave a little after nine. I'd do that every night. My father would often ask me to sit down and talk with him. I would tell him that I had to get the "stuff" done and there really wasn't time for talking.
>
> One day when I was driving home, I had a sudden awareness that I had gotten caught up in the routine "doing" and had been ignoring a limited opportunity to just be with my father and to share his thoughts and feelings. My new awareness drastically changed my caregiving routine. I got helpers in my father's house to do most of the needed daily chores, and I spent many hours with my father sharing conversations during the remainder of his life. I would listen and he would talk. My father wanted me to tell me about his values and what he had accomplished. He reminisced about his childhood, his parents, and how he grew up in the old country. He talked about his mother whom he last saw when he was

a child. He knew he was dying and would be with his deceased wife and his mother again soon.

My dad was a really deep thinker and a philosopher. Listening to him I had entered another level of our relationship, a kind of intimacy we'd never had before. Looking back, the illness I had damned for so long had, in truth, offered me a new way to be with my dad. Without his dependency on me and my participation in his care, I might never have experienced or understood what I came to learn, and I hope I never forget it.

I've come to understand that when we serve as caregivers, we, like this storyteller, often put all our energy and time into the practical things. Preparing and serving meals, making doctor appointments, tending to laundry, cleaning, running errands, and managing other necessities become our immediate concerns. The caregiver's schedule is often overloaded and exhausting. We seldom think we have time left for a cup of tea and conversation, a walk together in the garden, or just sitting quietly with an arm around the person in our care. As the story above shows, sharing conversations with the person in our care can be valuable in a variety of ways. Time spent talking and listening can offer both the caregiver and the person in care the opportunity to build a yet unexplored, deep, and meaningful level of exchange. Creating such connections often changes the life of the person now serving as the caregiver and without a question enriches each day of those in our care.

Although I heard this story from the caregiver's point of view, it left me wondering what the father might have said if I had also talked with him. That curiosity inspired me to assemble this new collection of stories giving voice to those who receive care.

In talking with several people now requiring some level of care,

I've learned how valuable deep, personal conversations, whether with the caregiver or with close relatives and friends, can be for a person receiving care. Care receivers often find substantive conversation as healing as medications. They might talk about memories and experiences, their current priorities and personal values, or the importance to them of spiritual or religious supports. For others a conversation can sometimes be a time of forgiveness and a healing of family separations and differences.

Often people in care may be eager to discuss even their impending death. That subject is not easy for some people to face and may be deliberately avoided in many families. Often, relief and comfort result from loved ones talking about death and other difficult subjects, what some have labeled "end of life issues," that need to be carefully detailed in writing to prevent survivor misunderstandings. A certified document in addition to a legal will covering finances, property, and other possessions can specify funeral arrangements, ceremonies, and other personal wishes and requests.

Those in recovery from an amputation, disabling injury, or the knowledge that permanent changes in lifestyle pose future limitations require honest conversation for return to a more normal activity level. Sometimes such realities aren't honestly faced by either the caregiver or the person in care. Yet, to reenter a meaningful life, possibly now with limitations, requires compromises and creative solutions that need to be openly and honestly considered.

Some people who share their stories in this book are dealing with a terminal disease, others an accident, a new disability, or a lifelong condition requiring continued care and resulting in a life of partial dependency. The stories cover a wide range of ages, from persons in their twenties up into their nineties. Many shared their thoughts and feelings, struggles and adjustments. Here are a couple of excerpts from a few of the stories you'll soon read.

- "It all goes back to what my mother taught me. This cancer is something I can't change. I can only deal with how I handle it, the attitude I bring into each day. Now, every day I remember my mother's philosophy. It's not just what happens to you but how you choose to live with it."

- "So many things that used to be so important don't really matter to me anymore. I always wanted things I couldn't afford. . . . They've become small things to me. The way I look at the world now has changed drastically. I look back, and I'm grateful for everything I've had and for the days ahead that I will have."

- "Death doesn't scare me, but . . . I want my family and friends and all those I've worked with and lived with in my lifetime to remember what my life stood for. . . . I want to think that I've left a legacy of fighting for justice and social equity, . . . and I hope many others will pick up where I've left off."

- "I am going to keep loving my life no matter what comes along. I have no complaints. I'm thankful for all the love and support that has kept me going and made it possible for me to get through the challenges of these many days. I've learned that the healing journey takes patience and courage and hope. Here's to more wonderful days! I'm in a place of peace."

All the persons in care I talked with wanted me to share their story. Whatever care they needed, they wanted to pass on what they had learned about accepting their situation, how they had dealt with and adapted to new limitations, and the priorities they had set for themselves. Their stories tell about how their world has grown smaller and of their desire to reach into the larger world. Yet their view of what living each day means is bigger for them in a way they could not have imagined. Of course, not only those in our care grow in their understanding of life's challenges and rewards. All of us, whether we're the caregiver or the recipient of the care, also might one day have an opportunity to tell a story that talks about how either receiving or providing care can nurture our spirits and transform our lives.

Perhaps some readers will find the stories in this book merely interesting, but for others, some aspect of a tale might be life changing. In either case, whether you're the one receiving care or the one who has taken on the responsibilities of the caregiver, each person's story can offer pathways toward a more meaningful connection with self and another. While our society has begun paying attention to the experiences and challenges faced by those who provide care for family members, we do not often hear these voices of the cared for—persons who are frequently invisible participants in our busy world. These stories illuminate the trials, frustrations, hopes, and fears that reflect the thoughts of those in care as they learn to accept help and adjust to the changes and challenges in their lives.

Many years ago I came across a short quote in a children's book entitled *Crow and Weasel*. Author Barry Lopez writes, "If stories come to you, care for them, and learn to give them away where they are needed. Sometimes a person needs a story more than food to stay alive." My hope is that through the stories in this book, you will find this truth: both caregiving and receiving care come with hope and heartbreak for all of us. Yet to live each day fully and to be as present as possible is the joy of life each of us can discover.

TASHA
I CAME TO BELIEVE I COULD

Most people live and die with their music still unplayed. They never dare to try. —MARY KAY ASH

TASHA, A CHARMING AND INSPIRING WOMAN IN HER MIDTHIRTIES, is unable to walk and will never be able to do so, yet I'm sure she would agree with Mary Kay Ash's quotation that many will live their life without exploring their potential. Tasha was recently the keynote speaker at the annual meeting of a local caregiving organization and delivered her lively presentation while sitting comfortably in her wheelchair. This was one of many speeches she's been asked to deliver since her name became well known a few years ago, when the Mayo Clinic nominated her for the 2012 National Rehabilitation Champion Award. She also was recently named Ms. Wheelchair USA. But it's her story, and I'm going to let her tell it.

I was in my midteens, in high school, still living with my parents, enjoying being in rehearsals for a play when I had a terrible accident. I took one step backward on the stage and fell sixteen feet through a trapdoor. I landed on my head, my neck was broken, and my spinal cord was crushed. I was diagnosed as a quadriplegic and told I'd never walk again. I'm now paralyzed and have no feeling or movement from my chest down, and all ten of my fingers are paralyzed. I am going to be completely dependent and using a wheelchair for the rest of my life. This all happened eighteen years ago. It was as if my life ended before my adult life even began.

I have the most amazing family. They stood by me and encouraged me while they were struggling themselves with anxiety and depression, figuring out how this was going to affect the rest of their lives, and mine. For one thing, they had to sell the only home I had ever lived in. Our house was old, built 115 years ago, and not compatible for a wheelchair. It just couldn't be modified. Yet in spite of their own challenges, my family was there for me and has given me so much support.

I spent six months in the hospital, and while I was there, I met a young guy who was in a wheelchair. He couldn't walk at all, but he would often come and visit me. I never knew if he was a doctor or a patient or someone just assigned to visit people. He always had a smile on his face. He offered me a positive attitude, one I then adopted in spite of my limitations. For over a month after I left the hospital, I was in a residence with other kids in recovery. Most of them always had a smile on their face. They were happy, and there didn't seem to be any sign of depression in these kids. That experience helped me realize I had a choice about my attitude. I knew I could sit home and feel sorry for myself, but I honestly knew that wasn't going to help me in any way at all.

The year ahead for me at home was my senior year of high school. It was a year of struggle to hold on to a positive outlook. Yet I knew if I didn't hang on to that point of view, the reality of my situation would drag me down. I could see that people in the community and also my family expected me to be dependent the rest of my life. My healing wasn't a one-night miracle. I didn't just wake up one morning and find I was a happy person. But slowly I came around to truly understanding how many blessings I have in this life.

About a year or a little more after my accident, a friend invited me to go with her to see a play. Somehow that play showed me that a spirit of hope was out there, a support, something bigger than me. After seeing that play I could feel something inside me changing. I had always gone to church on Sunday with my family, but I wasn't religious at all. Whether you call it religious inspiration or whatever, I knew from my experience watching that play I could help others. I felt a peace in my heart from that night on, and it changed everything for me.

My friends believed in me, and new friends I made when I went to college were supportive and really great. So many genuinely cared for me, and I'm still close to many of them. I lived on campus, and I hired students to come in to care for me. They came in shifts. I depended on people I didn't know and had to trust they would turn up and help me. I kept changing what I was going to focus on in college, and nothing I tried seemed the right choice. I went to talk to one professor whom I had taken a course from in communication studies. He asked me what I wanted to do, and I kept saying that I really didn't know. He said, "Possibly you could be an inspirational speaker."

That suggestion didn't make sense to me at that moment, as I had never considered doing anything like that. Over the next few weeks, though, I often thought about what he had said to me.

I knew for sure I wanted to help people. One day I realized that speaking and giving people inspiration and hope was exactly how I could help others. I knew I could tell them how I had dealt with my challenges and held on to as much independence as possible. I also could tell them how I've learned to accept the help I need. The hardest part of my life is that I will always need to rely on getting help from others. I can't transfer myself in and out of bed or get into my wheelchair without help. I can't get dressed or get into or out of a chair by myself. My caregivers are a huge part of my life. I still have all my caregivers come in shifts. If people come late, then I'm late for everything in my day. I've had to develop patience. Other people are my hands, they're my body, and I've learned to accept the way they do things and be thankful that I have the help.

I can write on my computer, because it's voice activated. I've learned how to put a dish in the refrigerator and take it out. If there's a full meal on a plate, I can manage mealtime by myself. My life is a lot more independent than the doctors predicted when I had the accident. They prepared me for the worst, so every bit of independence I can develop is a victory. Others have taught me how to do things, and some things I've been able to figure out for myself.

My boyfriend stayed with me for a few months after the accident, but we broke up. The change was too much for him to handle. When I turned twenty-one, I made the decision that I wasn't going to try to find a husband until I felt I understood myself. I first had to be happy and confident being me. I actually went about ten years without dating anyone. I met some nice guys, but I needed to be comfortable with myself.

I wanted to come and go as I pleased. I wanted to have time alone and be comfortable with that.

I often spoke to groups at businesses, churches, and my own church. I wasn't speaking full time. I traveled all over with a caregiver or my mom or my sister. I didn't let anything hold me back. If I needed two people to come with me to help, I'd hire two people, simple as that.

I knew my mom would always be there for me. She put up with a lot from me. In the past, I took a lot of frustration out on her. I know she would never leave me, but others would if I gave them a hard time. My mom still fills in if I need someone in a pinch, but that's very rare. I'm fortunate now to live in a house that is built to accommodate my needs.

When I turned thirty I began trying online dating. I didn't really want to do it, but my girlfriend insisted. Ironically, that's how I met my husband, Doug. We were on e-mail and Skype for hours. I don't think he ever had known someone in a wheelchair. He used to work as a meteorologist. Now we work together, and he does all the things I don't like to do—the spreadsheets, billing, budgeting, and the paperwork. I only do the speaking; that's my passion. Every group I speak to is different. Some people are young, some older, some are having troubled times, some are ill, some are caring for others. I enjoy talking to them all.

My husband wanted to help people. I guess in some ways we have the same goals. We decided together that he wasn't going to be my caregiver. His job was to be my husband. I want to have a healthy marriage. It was the best decision in our now over one year of being married. When we go on a trip together, that is the one time when he's my caregiver for a short period. That has worked fine, and we have a good time.

What difference do my caregivers make in my day? The way

I deal with my caregivers affects my whole life. We laugh, we joke, and my caregivers become my friends. Last month I spoke eleven times in five days. One of my caregivers went on the trip with me. She heard me give almost the same speech every time. She was amazing. Two days we had to get up at five in the morning and we were out until eleven o'clock at night. I was so glad she was with me. The schedule was rigorous, but she was fun, and that made it a good experience. My caregivers make a huge difference in my life.

I'm thankful every day that I held on during the tough times. This is my life now, and I tell you honestly that I wouldn't change it. I talk with teenagers who have thought about suicide. Each group I now speak to, both young and old, in care or giving care, I have an open time for personal sharing after my talk. I have to trust that something I share with individuals or groups will help people find the courage to deal with whatever problem they're facing. I hope my work can leave a legacy in the world that fear and depression can be overcome.

When I speak at a conference or with a group, I want to believe that if one life is touched, if a person is motivated to heal, then it's meant to be. That's what I continue to do, in my way, to inspire others to help live a better life. I can see when I speak that my story means something important for some people. A look on their faces tells me that. I talk to women's groups about how to accept themselves and love themselves as they are. I want people to find the person they are at whatever age or stage of life they're at. We look at the images in magazines, and we know we don't fit that model. Many older women have fears and complaints about getting old. I remind them that some people never get the option of living to an old age.

Now, thankfully, as we're having this conversation, it's twenty-six years since my accident, and sometimes I forget that I'm in a wheelchair. This is now my new normal, and I love my life. To sit home and feel sorry for myself is pointless. I can go out and help others and bring inspiration into this world for many who need a boost to help themselves. I had to be my biggest cheerleader. People told me for so many years that I couldn't, I wouldn't, I shouldn't, but I came to believe I could. I give it everything I have. I don't offer any particular message in my speaking except to live with purpose, and that's what I hope to help others find for themselves. I live my story.

> *I believe in the power of stories to dismantle boundaries, build community, and offer healing words to someone open to hearing them.*
> —AN ANONYMOUS FAMILY CAREGIVER

There are times in all our lives when the path ahead might seem hopeless. To keep from sinking further into hopelessness and helplessness can be the biggest and most important challenge of a lifetime. Some people in my life by just their presence, their words, their attitude, and their smile, have helped me hang on as I found my life-affirming path. As you read this book, you probably will recall such times in your life or in the lives of others who needed you to just hold their hands during stormy times.

Each of us can get personal inspiration and new insights from unexpected sources. The words, the stories of someone of a different age, religion, or race, or who is dealing with a totally different problem, may surprisingly offer us the information or inspiration we're searching to find for ourselves. Possibly the grit and determination of the way Tasha has accepted her limitations and taken on the challenges to build her life around them may give us or someone we know a gift of possible independence. Limitations are not always limitations.

1. Share your story or one from others you know about positive change growing out of a negative situation or new limitation.

2. What public lecture or group event offered you an unexpected insight, a challenging point of view, or an idea that changed your philosophy that led you to make new choices?

3. Have you ever discovered or helped someone else understand that a victim attitude doesn't serve us well? If so, what new awareness did you help that person discover? What did you learn as a result of that experience?

DAVID
ACCEPTANCE AND CONTENTMENT

> *When you have decided what you believe, what you feel must be done, have the courage to stand alone and be counted.* —ELEANOR ROOSEVELT

SOME GIFTS DON'T COME WRAPPED IN PRETTY PAPER WITH A fancy bow. My friend David has given me the gift of some unusual reflections on living and dying and his view of caregiving. He was my friend for more than thirty years. We supported and encouraged each other as our careers developed, and as each of our philosophies and knowledge in the field of aging grew and deepened.

His perspective and passion are reflected in books he wrote throughout his career: *Firms of Endearment, Ageless Marketing,* and *Serving the Ageless Market.* During the few years when David's health was deteriorating, he captured his passion for elders by writing yet another book about the American view of aging, *Brave New Worldview*. The manuscript was finished the day a group of friends who knew David's work and philosophy came to his home to help him complete the final chapters. When they raised their glasses of champagne to celebrate, David smiled and shared his satisfaction, although he couldn't share the bubbly. His death came a few days later.

I had recorded my last conversation with David just a few weeks earlier. That day, before I gave David a last hug, I asked, "May I share your words with others?" "Yes, of course," he answered. And I replied, "I was counting on that!" He knew he was facing death, yet he talked about living, continuing to learn, and how much he valued his wife, who was now his caregiver, and his attentive family and his many friends. Here are some reflections he shared with me.

I'm seventy-seven now. I was diagnosed with lung cancer three years ago, and that's now in stage 4. I also have an aortic aneurysm and an edema in my left leg. I have atrial fibrillation, and I've had chronic lymphedema for about fifteen years. My life is almost totally governed by the medical community and all these ailments that I have. My periodic excursions to the hospital come fairly often now, and the timing of those is out of my control. I remember one week when it all got to be too much—seeing a second doctor, a third doctor, and then a fourth doctor. I came away from that episode realizing that to the medical community, I'm a machine that isn't in good working shape. I know parts of me need to be fixed, but realistically I know that goal is impossible. They're not going to be able to fix me. So, I let the doctors do their job, taking care the best they can of those physical things, and I'll take care of the rest of my life.

Do I think about death? I've thought about it often during the past fifteen years, since I was diagnosed with lymphatic cancer. When I got the diagnosis of stage 4 lung cancer, I don't think I was really surprised. I'd been living for years with the warnings of a doctor who told me that my cancer made me more subject to other cancers. I'm not threatened by loss of independence. I'm beyond harm's way. I'm living in the ever-present present. I live today and don't let a fear of dying get in the way of my desire to enjoy this day. I live with living, not dying.

My youngest daughter was eight years old at the time of my original diagnosis, and I remember thinking that staying around at least until she was through high school was important to me. I was divorced, and there wasn't a woman around the house. One day my daughter said to me, "Dad, maybe it's time for you to get married again. I'm about to become a woman," she said emphatically, "and I need a woman around." So, I started dating. When I started seeing Linda a lot, I told her about my diagnosis in one breath and asked her to marry me in the next. Now we've been married for seventeen years.

People are important in my life. I have family who come to see me often, but I'm substantially dependent on Linda for almost everything. My dependence on her involves my co-operation and acceptance of my dependency. She deserves the satisfaction of knowing that her efforts make a difference for me. I think I've become pretty responsive to her needs. I just instinctively knew that the harder I made it for Linda, the more I risked her feeling regretful and resentful about my situation. I've worked constantly on my attitude and feel no loss of dignity when I can no longer do things I've always been able to do for myself.

It's a very important thing to be aware when you're in someone's care that you can actually make things harder for the caregiver. I have a friend who is so obsessed with maintaining his independence that he makes it hard on everyone around him who offers help. He should really use a cane, because he's not steady and often falls. He can't drive anymore, and he constantly complains about that. He's gone into a stage of some necessary dependence, and he's done it without any grace. He doesn't seem to realize that with such behavior you can wear out a caregiver and injure yourself.

Here's how I see things. We value our independence so much in this culture that we tend to think of dependence as weakness. People who are embittered, angry, or ill-tempered, but who need others to care for them, often are dreadfully unhappy. They make their situation worse by projecting their unhappiness onto their caregiver. I've become far less focused on maintaining a myth of independence, which so many ill people feel is a major accomplishment.

My dependency doesn't prevent me from finding meaning in life. I can't go out on the basketball court, but I can think and write about my ideas and thoughts. I don't know if I'll be leaving my wife financially secure enough, but I can't do anything to change the present situation. When I look ahead to the future, I'm confident my kids are all in great shape. They're in good marriages, and they're in fairly secure financial shape. I have a loving and attentive family, and those relationships are important to me. My grandchildren love me. I'm told that even their dog gets excited when my daughter says, "We're going to Grandpa's house." So, I haven't lost my feelings of worth.

I have a sense of value because of what I'm writing and working on each day. I may not be able to dance these days, but I still have a sense that the words I write can make the world dance. When I look at my future, I think about finishing the book I'm writing. I feel I have something important to say about my belief that as we become more and more technologically dependent, we've become less human.

My new book will be entitled *Brave New Worldview*. I believe we are trying to make sense of a worldview that took root in Newtonian science more than three centuries ago, the view that the universe is a giant clockwork-like mechanism. Over time, the whole of society embraced this mechanistic view. Human properties such as empathy, creativity, emotions, and spiritual essence are increasingly written off as corruptors of that "truth." I feel compelled to write about what I believe is the loss of this human truth. I have a personal mission to say these things, particularly to people working in advertising and marketing who so often define us humans as atrophied. We are now valued more for the technology we create than for the gifts of mind and spirit that make technology and its relentless advance possible.

Genuine personal interaction does not happen on Twitter, Facebook, or e-mail. My grandson said something to me jokingly the other day: "Twitter is for people who don't have a life to communicate with people who don't have a life!" I've found that communication through a computer is not the preferred grandparent-grandchild interaction. Yes, there's Skype, the system that allows you to see the other person. I guess it's better than nothing, but it's not the real thing.

The point I want to get across in my new book is that thirty-year-olds and younger people who now are creating advertising have no idea what our aging American society is about. They aren't presenting age authentically. They too often think that older people should work toward being forever young. It's offered as the only truth. Stay young, and that will carry you through your conversations, your work, and your entire life. Movies, advertising, and much in our society continues to promote an unrealistic picture of older persons. Look around. You'll see seventy-three million baby boomers aging and trying desperately to stay young! I have a more realistic vision, and my book will present that. This is what keeps me going, although I well know that I'm getting weaker each day.

I'm often asked where I get my inspiration or comfort. Some people facing death have a very large concern about what happens to us after our death. Others look to a religious belief that promises something specific after death. Many find solace in the idea that they're leaving behind something worthwhile, their life work, and that they'll live on forever through that. My point of view isn't really any of those. I just look at today. I get my inspiration from what I'm doing at the moment, not a final prize. I've looked back on my youth and remembered poor relationships with my teachers, my unpopularity as a child, and that I never had many friends. I had a negative vision of the world. I know myself better now than I have during all the rest of my life. At my stage of life I don't need to be defined by other people. I've made peace with myself.

If could say anything meaningful to people who are dealing with what we label a terminal illness, I'd tell them to make a decision to take negativism out of their consciousness. I've found that by accomplishing that, everything else falls into place. This doesn't mean that I live without judgment; I recognize that bad things happen in the world. Yet in my personal life, I've managed to take negativism out of my conscious vocabulary, and consequently I've still been developing and evolving. I've found that if past negative experiences and judgments about myself no longer exist for me, then only a positive attitude toward myself is present.

I didn't get to this place automatically. I've been through a process of deep learning. Each of us as we face multiple challenges in our lives can, at any age or stage of life, continue to grow. Several people I know who have been diagnosed with a fatal illness have talked with me about how living with their awareness of death has brought them to a transcendent stage—to a deeper, higher awareness. This state of mind that I'm talking about takes them—and maybe me too—to a higher state of being.

I recently heard a quote I've come to believe is true: "Dying is our last developmental act." We don't know how to die. For so many of us, it scares us, intimidates us. We become resentful and bitter. You can't read a how-to book on dying. Rather, our best learning can actually come from ourselves. Each of us is given the opportunity to figure out our own way. It's an internal journey, a personal one. I'm on mine now, and I'm very much at peace. I know I can't live much longer, but I'm hopeful my ideas will live on.

> ***Decide that each day will be good just because you are here, that you will live life to the fullest now, no matter what.*** —ANONYMOUS

David and many others tell us, in their own way, that embracing the reality of death can enrich each day of their life. Our mortality need not be the daily focus of our lives, however. The richness and beauty of life is found in how we live it even when we're truly aware that our time in this life is limited. Not only philosophers, but also many ordinary people are comfortable telling us in their own words that death is a part of everyone's life. They remind us to live our lives as fully as each day allows. We don't necessarily have to be faced with a terminal illness to come to a place of peace within ourselves. Death is part of life for all living creatures. Accepting that reality can truly enrich each of our days and give meaning and value to a small experience as well as a major accomplishment.

Another insight and gift to us in David's story relates to caregiving. David was well aware that the caregiving responsibilities and burdens on his wife became more and more challenging. While I was at his home and he made requests for help, I observed that he was concerned for and considerate of Linda. I saw David offer her a word of thanks, a smile of gratitude, a squeeze of her hand. He offered her the gift of appreciation and nourishing support.

At a conference I recently attended, one speaker talked about the term *caregiver.* He pointed out that the word implies one person is the giver of care, and the job of the other is to receive the care. He suggested a possible change of perspective—that caregiving is not about one person taking charge of everything while another person loses his or her independence. Rather, it's about both people becoming partners in care. He encouraged the audience to use the phrase *care partner* and to adopt an attitude and perspective consistent with that term. Becoming care partners is a cooperation that can reduce the feelings of loss.

1. Those being cared for need to experience all the independence that is safe and possible for them. Describe a situation in which you or someone you have observed have allowed a person receiving care to act independently in appropriate situations.

2. When, and in what ways, have you as a caregiver or someone you've observed not allowed a person to act independently or possibly not recognized that he or she was able to do so?

3. What experience have you had talking with someone about the reality and acceptance of his or her impending death? How has that conversation unfolded? What did you learn from it?

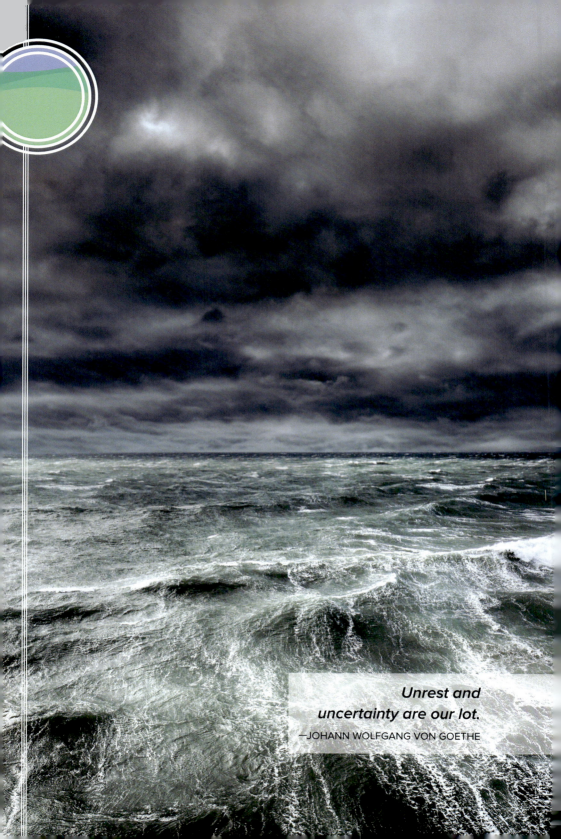

> Unrest and uncertainty are our lot.
> —JOHANN WOLFGANG VON GOETHE

JULIE
HE'S WITH ME FOR THE JOURNEY

THE WORDS DEMENTIA AND ALZHEIMER'S DISEASE ARE FRIGHT-ening to many people and may be giving you a reason to turn the page and skip Julie's story. Please don't leave before Julie and her husband, Tom, share their story of love, commitment, inspiration, and hope.

Although Julie has a specific diagnosis, a lot of people with memory problems have had no formal diagnosis, or they have some other dementia or problems related to forgetting. Researchers say about 30 percent of people who have dementia do not have Alzheimer's. It's important to understand that not all dementia is Alzheimer's. It's only one of a number of possible causes of dementia and memory loss.

One day a neighbor of mine told me about Julie, who had recently received a diagnosis of early onset Alzheimer's. I made a plan to visit Julie, and she greeted me at the door with a smile. Without hesitation, Julie opened our conversation with these words: "You want me talk to about my memory problems and how our lives have changed, right?" Yes, she was right, and I was hoping too that Julie would tell me about plans they were making to deal with the future. She began our conversation with the story of her and her husband's long relationship.

I'm fifty-seven years old, I have two children, and I've been married thirty years—oh, it's maybe thirty-seven. I don't actually remember. My husband, Tom, and I met in high school. We were both in the school band and both played trumpet. He had a cute way of taking his mouthpiece out of his mouth, and he would blow me kisses. We were around fourteen or fifteen years old. I'm Lutheran, and he's Catholic, and my parents would say things like, "It's nice that you have a friendship," but what they really meant was that if I was going to get serious, I should find my own kind.

When we graduated from high school, I went off to college and he went to—I don't remember, but it was maybe some state university or a Catholic college. We eventually were married, and we moved to where he could finish his studies and graduate. Then we moved somewhere else that I don't remember, but where I could go to nursing school. When I graduated, we moved to a location where Tom got a good job as an accountant.

I don't specifically remember when my memory began to give me problems. I was a busy person out in the world and had started my own business called Catalyst for Sustainable Change. It grew out of my nursing training, which helped me understand what diagnosing and giving care require. It taught me how to help others move from unhealth to health and greater clarity. I was also trained as a community mediator. My training and experience in those two fields provided the philosophy underlying my business. I know that I helped others, and I loved my work.

Consulting requires listening very carefully, taking what

I've heard and putting all the pieces together very quickly. In my work, I moved from many obvious and subtle clues toward solutions. I remember when I was beginning to become aware—for two, maybe three, maybe even five years—that my ability to put those pieces together was becoming limited. I just couldn't do it easily or well anymore.

Then one day I noticed I was beginning to take hours to get a presentation together. It was something that used to take me no time at all. But I'd work a half a day on reorganizing my materials, and then I'd find that they were actually back in their original order. I've always been a competent, independent person, and it all just came to me easily. Now I'm not that person. The changes were gradual, and then I just wasn't that me anymore.

My husband started to realize how long simple tasks were taking me. I tried to relax about the changes and not get anxious, but I felt I wasn't functioning right. Simple things were getting me confused. We scheduled an appointment with a reputable neurologist, and I went though a series of tests, memory games, and other diagnostic steps. When Tom and I heard the words *early-onset Alzheimer's,* we walked silently out of the doctor's office. We sat in the car, held on to each other, and both cried.

Very soon after the diagnosis we began to reorganize our lives. I've had to leave my job. We're making a plan to sell the home we live in now and move into an apartment. Tom has taken on the responsibility of caretaker of the apartment building where we're going to be living, so he can have more time at home with me. Tom will be doing maintenance in the apartment complex, and that will give us a much lower rent. We talked together about his doing that and made the decision together. His love for me, his deep spiritual feelings, and his desire to give me the care I need now and will need more in the future are the reasons he's left his position. Tom is making this change with love.

My parents strongly disapprove. They think he should hold on to his job and his paycheck and that someone else should take care of me. He's taken a lot of criticism and anger from both of our families for his decision to leave his job and take on the responsibility of my care. But this change in our living situation is what we decided we both want. Tom is giving me the gift of himself, and for some reason that seems to be hard for both sets of parents to accept.

Months after my original conversation with Julie, the mutual friend who had originally suggested I contact Julie told me that she and her husband, Tom, had sold their home and were settled in an apartment, as they had planned. I contacted Tom to set up another appointment to talk with Julie. He told me that the move had been somewhat difficult for her and that getting familiar and comfortable in their new surroundings was challenging. Julie recognized me when I arrived for our second conversation, however.

I'll tell you about my life now. You can see we've moved out of our house and into this apartment. My husband, Tom, takes care of this whole building. Now that he left his job, he doesn't have to go away to work anymore. He's always here by my side or in the building. I know that his caring and wisdom will support me as my Alzheimer's progresses. He's very spiritually reflective and meditates and prays every morning. Even though we came from different religious backgrounds, our once separate practices and philosophies have come together.

The hardest thing for me now is to fill up a day. I used to be so busy and connected to work and other people. I take a walk every morning on paths I know, so I can get back easily. I go to a yoga class twice a week, and I like to knit. I like to watch television. When we watch a longer television program together, I write down questions about things I'm confused about, and I ask Tom to answer during the commercials. I often can't remember the beginning of the show we're watching, and I need help to sometimes understand the end of a TV drama. These days it takes a lot longer to read a book. I like mysteries, and I most often can't remember what the beginning part of the book was. I have to go back and read pieces of the beginning and then the middle again. I experience other memory lapses throughout the day.

My children are adults; they're thirty-one and twenty-nine. My older son works for a company that's researching how to use lasers and computations to figure out solutions for a variety of challenges and problems. He's also doing everything he can to research new ways of understanding and dealing with Alzheimer's. He's attempting to work with people who do that research, hoping he can be part of finding a cure for my kind of dementia.

I have one grandchild who is almost three. He lives with his parents here in the city where we live and comes to visit every other Friday. I can't take care of him alone now, but we've arranged for different friends of mine to come over and be here with us.

My doctor keeps telling me to exercise every day, and he sent me to yoga because when I do yoga, my head is often down and I guess it's good for the blood to go to my head. He often reminds me to do what I want to do and can do. I take one medication, Aricept. It's a drug that slows the formation of plaque that forms around some of the brain cells.

Tom and I go together to a class for early onset Alzheimer's patients. One man there couldn't use his hands at all, and another couldn't speak. The biggest discussion that goes on in that group is "Can you drive? How long will you drive? What will you do when you can't drive?"

One day when I was driving to yoga, I got lost. Since then I've used a GPS system for everything, so I just follow what it tells me to do. I don't know at this point how long I'll be able to follow those directions. I'm going to try hard to hold on to what I can still do.

My friends can't really believe, or don't want to believe, that someone my age has Alzheimer's. They don't have the experience or understanding to figure out some of my behaviors. I'm having trouble with that too. Some of my casual friends aren't around much anymore, but my longtime friends are there for me. I have the friends I feel I need. I've always felt like I have to do everything myself, so I'm still uncomfortable with everyone doing things for me, but I know that accepting their help is what I need to do. I continue to experience a loss of capabilities, but my biggest fear is that I've started to experience the loss of myself. I'm frightened of being frightened. I don't know what I won't know. That's the best and the worst thing about my diagnosis.

Tom and I talk regularly about what I'm now having trouble doing by myself and what I need help with. I'm still able to have intelligent, two-way conversations about such things. My husband and I are having a really huge role reversal. I used to be the one in charge, and now I'm not capable of that anymore. Tom is pretty much in charge now, and I'm not used to that yet. I can't believe my husband, who I thought was so dependent upon me, is now strong and confident and taking care of me. We cry together, and he holds me. That comfort and closeness is so important for me.

I still know how to do some things, but now I can't do other things at all. I wanted to write a letter on my computer. I couldn't remember how to do it. My husband showed me how, and then I wanted to send it but couldn't remember how to do that. I have to ask for so many things now. I've been a very independent and a very competent person. Now I hope those around me can be there for me and help with kindness and understanding.

I've had to give up a lot of things, and I'll have to give up more in the days to come. I know I just have to keep going. I'm not depressed, but I'm sad about what I've lost already and what I will lose in the future. It's hard for me to think about this. Many people out there are thinking of me, praying for me, and doing things for me. I've come to a place of feeling comfortable about accepting what people offer. I have a loving husband, and my children are concerned and present, and I know they'll all be there for me as my life becomes more and more constricted. I can't look too far ahead. I just have to deal with every day. Alzheimer's wasn't in my plan, but that's the way it turned out.

I know and now accept that it's time for others to take care of me.

Almost three years after my first conversation with Julie, I scheduled a telephone conversation with Julie's husband, Tom. I wanted to follow up on each of them before this book was finished. Tom carefully plans his work schedule and home time with Julie. He's now able to go to work three days a week. He counsels and offers support to people who see him at a spiritual education service. On those days, Julie goes to a day program for people with memory loss. Her deteriorated condition is less severe than some in the class, and her leadership abilities have surfaced and are helpful for both her and others in the group. She actively interacts in the group and with the leaders themselves. She's actually taken on a partial leadership role. Tom says that it enriches Julie's experience and builds her confidence. The group has organized a choir, and they often perform at various nursing homes and other venues in the community. Music has enriched those who perform, as well as their audiences.

Julie stays at home some days and has visits that Tom schedules with relatives; her grandchildren—ages six and four years, and nine months; friends; and others who schedule times to be with Julie. Tom has hired various helpers to do some of the necessary cleaning and laundry. The days Tom spends at home with Julie include going to a health club together. They can walk there directly through their backyard. Because her memory for getting to once-familiar locations is gone, Julie has had to give up driving. Television watching is more comfortable with Tom than alone, because Tom can help her with the continuity of the program.

Tom told me that Julie cries more often. One of her friends in the day program passed away recently, and it brought on crying sessions for many days. Other sad experiences that brought Julie to tears were losing the capacity to drive, recently much reduced physical mobility, and her awareness that her loss of skills continues at a quickened pace. Although she often tells Tom that she feels like a child when others need to tell her what to do and when, she's greatly empowered by the memory-loss group, because she's found a role there that allows her to help others. Tom believes the living and working arrangements they developed together have kept Julie more confident and relatively calm and accepting. In his words, "We're partners in this challenge."

> *Life is not about waiting*
> *for the storms to pass;*
> *it's about learning to dance*
> *in the rain.* —VIVIAN GREENE

In 2017, as the medical world seeks to find both the causes and a possible cure, nearly 5.5 million people in the United States have Alzheimer's disease or some other dementia. Many of us have relatives, friends, neighbors, or colleagues who have such a disease and have shared at least some aspect of Tom and Julie's experience.

A diagnosis of Alzheimer's disease is sure to be a life challenge. No one behavior or specific symptom defines the disease or other dementia. Each person who is living with dementia acts and responds differently, and has unique needs and varied effects on his or her primary caregivers. Some people with dementia are very aware of every change and loss. Others enter a deteriorated stage not understanding their decline and unaware of the consequences of their unpredictable actions. We all know about people with an Alzheimer's diagnosis who experience uncontrollable behavior, wander out of the house, and can be unpredictable and even violent. Ultimately dementia results in drastic changes for the person with dementia and all those around him or her.

The experience of family caregivers differs from one situation to another, but dementia presents difficult and unexpected challenges as the disorder progresses. There often is no way to plan, because the rate of decline is individual and unpredictable. Often family and friends can do little besides sit with the person they are caring for and hold his or her hand. A caregiver or a person with dementia—I can't remember which—once said to me, "I handle each day best if I go with the flow." That simple phrase offers wisdom for both the person being cared for and the primary caregiver.

1. Families involved in providing care for people with Alzheimer's or other dementia make a variety of decisions about how to help loved ones. In situations you're aware of, who in the family has been involved in decision making? Are any decisions clearly right or wrong?

2. How has a diagnosis of Alzheimer's or another type of dementia touched your family or someone you've dealt with? What have you learned about memory loss, your coping skills, and yourself? How have you integrated those insights into your work or personal life?

3. Have you had any experience with support groups for persons with early-onset Alzheimer's? If so, was the support group helpful? What specific suggestions worked well? What didn't work? How might you approach caring for a loved one differently?

DIANNE
ENJOYING MY LIFE

The people you need to help you make your dream come true are everywhere and within your reach. —MARCIA WIEDER

I MET DIANNE A NUMBER OF YEARS AGO, WHEN I MOVED TO THE Midwest. She worked with the Area Agency on Aging as a regional planner and program consultant for twenty-four counties. She knew everything related to aging programs and services in the area. Because I was interested in aging and related subjects, we often met and talked about family caregiving and other concerns relating to older persons.

Our conversation during a recent visit was more personal than usual. During the past few months she had become quite different from the independent, energetic woman I met years ago. Although Dianne was only in her midfifties, she had metastatic adenocarcinoma of the appendix, the peritoneal cavity, and the vaginal wall. The cancer was rapidly spreading throughout her entire body, and now she was the one receiving care from family and others. Dianne was very aware that her days were numbered. She asked me to add her story to this book, as she wanted to tell people something that she had learned about life and now deeply felt. "Each morning when I wake up is a gift." Dianne wanted her words to live on.

I had been the regional planning agent for our Area Agency on Aging. Several regions merged, and now the agency I worked with serves seventy counties. I knew when I was diagnosed with cancer what the consequences would probably be. The job was nothing I could do anymore, as it meant driving all over the state. I wasn't choosing to leave my career of thirty-five years, but my contract wasn't renewed when I became ill. When the agency rejected me for my old job, it took me a while to realize that I'm bigger than their rejection. That realization gave me my voice back.

When I was at Mayo Clinic recovering from my colon surgery, I remember standing in the hall and seeing a woman leaning limply against a wall and crying. A doctor approached her, put her arms around her, and just held her. I felt an incredible heart connection to that episode, like my own heart came back alive, and I said to myself, "I must be about the work of the heart." The message was very strong, something I couldn't deny. I've now made my life mission helping goodness grow. I have time now to listen more. It's important to listen to what people care about. We all need to be heard.

Everything I've learned in the job I had I'm now trying to use, as I'm still able, to do and give, to contribute. I knew I had a mission. My life calling is to continue to improve the lives of people who are older, people with disabilities, and caregivers. It's still all the same work without the job title attached to it. I'm doing it in different ways by working as a volunteer with the End of Life Coalition and the Grief and Loss Center, and working on issues of caregiving and receiving care that were always a focus for me in my work. There's no paycheck with my self-defined job, but my reward is that I've got my voice. I've been doing advocacy with my state government and even the White House. I've written letters to the local newspaper editor. And I've spoken out on many issues related to senior care assistance, services for family caregivers, and other related areas. I have knowledge, connections, and experience. I've slowed up considerably in recent weeks, but when I feel that I can participate, I still do. I'm reaping the harvest from my life's work.

I'm also learning to be more open and honest with my own feelings than I've ever been able to be in my life. My becoming ill has opened the door to a whole different kind of learning for me. I'm very much in charge of my own care, yet I've learned how important it is to make a meaningful connection with those who are responsible for my care in the medical field. There's an art to engaging, as a person, a doctor and others who are responsible for my care. I've often written thank-you notes to my doctors when they've made a positive connection with me.

I've been telling you about my new understanding of the work I've been doing. As for my personal life, when I first was diagnosed with cancer, I made a list of things that I wanted to do and called it "Dianne's Amazing Future Life Adventures List." Now I've just completed my first year of living with delight. That's what I've called it. I did a bunch of the stuff on my list. My sister and I went to see Lake Superior in the winter. The sun was shining on big chunks of ice. It was beautiful. Then I wanted to get on the train and visit friends in Seattle and Portland I hadn't seen in thirty years. I did that right after I finished a dozen sessions of chemotherapy. While I was there I saw the mountains and the amazing ocean, and I went to Vancouver, British Columbia. I met so many interesting people on the train. I have more plans for train trips on my adventures list. I hope I'll be strong enough to take them.

I need to slow down now, to adopt a different pace in my life. These days I read and ponder. My life now is so different from the way I lived all the busy, active years. My approach is just to take one day at a time. Something in me is motivated to gather wisdom. I've spent these days in conversations I've been able to arrange with some counselors, psychologists, psychiatrists, and ministers who I've known. I've also always worked with older people, and I've collected many stories in which they've shared their wisdom. Now I live with the seeds of their inspiration.

I often think about my dad. He was a hardworking insurance man with eight mouths to feed. At the age of fifty he was diagnosed with heart failure. At that time, I immediately worked to change my relationship with him and clear up some tensions in our past. I closely watched how he adapted to changes in his life. On days when he wasn't well enough to work, he would sit and watch the birds. I remember how many times he said to me, "All this quiet except for the birds on the windowsill." I remember too that he would sit quietly and watch the patterns of the clouds and look with wonder at the night sky. When I was in graduate school I wrote to him every week, and he answered me. I remember one letter he wrote and asked me if I realized that there were fifty-three varieties of ants in our backyard. That's what you do when you're not able to do what you used to do. You sit and observe. His looking at the ants was actually a mindfulness practice. He swallowed the reality of his diagnosis, but he didn't retreat or withdraw. He lived his life as best he could, and that was my example to do the same. My father has inspired me to live fully the life I have left.

My hope for now is that I have an amazing summer of delight. I want to spend time with my daughters, my siblings, and my mom in Ohio, and I hope to gather longtime friends and enjoy them all. Every day I get cards, phone calls, and e-mails, and I feel valued. I don't know what the future holds, but one thing I do know is that in many ways I'm in the best place in my whole life. I don't know what's coming in the months ahead, but I know for sure that I won't be alone.

I have a great sense of peace about my life and a new understanding that there's so much beauty in every day. This has come to me through all the people I know, all over the world, who are praying for me and wishing for my healing in whatever way healing is meant to happen. I don't know if I'll live a long life, if I'll see much of the future or my grandchildren, but my spirit is quite whole. Strange to say, but while dealing with my cancer I've had a great healing of the spirit. It's all been a blessing.

> *I will think about the choices I make today and what they say about me as a person.* —LINDA PICONE

Dianne's story reveals that she accepts the reality of her medical condition. I admire her brave and wise actions in reaching out to people in her life. When people are faced with such diagnosis, they often succumb to their fears, going into depression and withdrawal. Those who deny instead of adapting to their new reality aren't fully living what life they may have left to live. We all have only now, this hour, this day. Dianne has actively engaged in each day in spite of the knowledge that her days are limited.

Another important aspect of Dianne's story for me was her affirmation that we need purposeful activity in our days. Dianne volunteered in a community and subject area she understands and cares about. I've talked with others who have found meaning for themselves in gardening, cooking a delicious meal, sharing memories with a friend or relative, meditation, prayer, or just enjoying a big breakfast. Meaning in each of our days can change based on our current circumstances. No activity, mental or physical, big or small, is too minor or unimportant if it has meaning for us.

Dianne reached out in her own behalf and made it easy for others to respond. Many of her old contacts, and new ones, responded to her phone calls, e-mails, postcards, and invitations to make plans. Making that effort isn't always easy or successful for the ill person, however. Well and busy people often feel they don't know how to be with or what to talk about with a person who is ill. Family members and friends sometimes need help understanding that the person they knew and enjoyed is still inside that changing body.

My conversation with Dianne motivated me to think about several encounters I've had with sick friends. I remember times when I visited ill friends or shared an activity of their choice at their pace. When they said, "Thank you so much for spending this afternoon with me," I sincerely replied, "No, let me thank you. It's been so good being with you." We most often get back more than we give. For me, and most probably for you, an interaction with others, well or ill, can greatly enrich our days.

We all know, or will know at some time in our lives, people who are dealing with some disease or disability that limits their lifestyle.

Many of my colleagues and friends are dealing with some ailment or diagnosis that has imposed limitations. I am actively trying to keep in touch with them, although our old activities together have changed. Whether you're dealing with personal limitations and changes or those of a friend, I hope Dianne's story will enrich and motivate you.

1. What stories can you share about a time when you have been attentive to your friends and relatives who have slowed down, limited their activity, or become housebound? Do you sometimes resist spending time with them? What have you learned that you can pass on to others?

2. The term *bucket list* (a list of things a person wishes to experience or accomplish before the end of his or her life) has become quite popular. How could you help someone you know, work with, or are caring for do some activity on his or her own bucket list?

3. What for you is the most powerful awareness you've experienced as a result of Dianne's story?

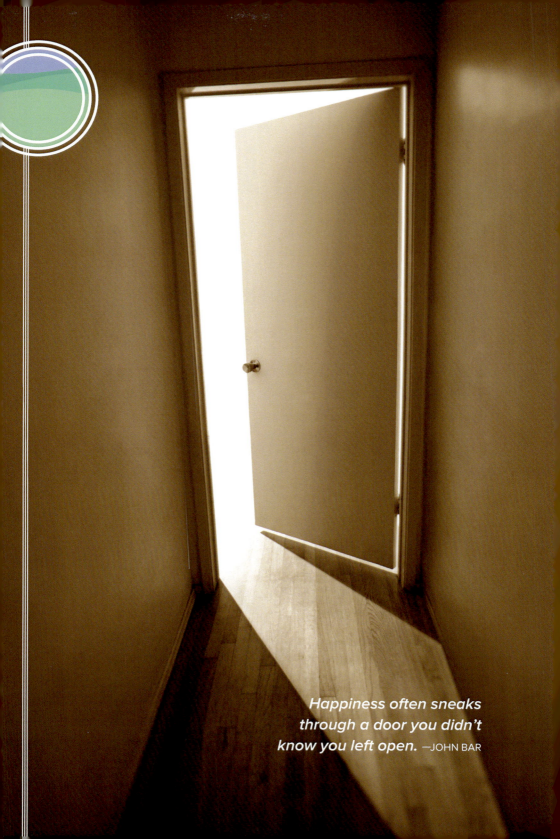

Happiness often sneaks through a door you didn't know you left open. —JOHN BAR

BETTY
I FOUND A NEW LIFE

I TALKED WITH BETTY SOON AFTER SHE HAD CELEBRATED HER ninetieth birthday. She's an outspoken elder who feels she has something to teach by the way she dealt with uninvited changes and challenges in her life. Her story is an inspiring tale of continuing to learn and grow out of her depression and feelings of helplessness into a limited but full life. Betty was eager to share her tale of woe and transition.

Once upon a time my life was very different from the way it is now. I've traveled a lot; I visited twenty-four countries during an era when you could travel cheaply and have a great adventure. For a few years I lived in Mexico, where I took up collage and developed a sort of a mini art career for a while before I moved back to the States. I had a busy and interesting life during my time in Mexico. I took classes, studied writing, and became involved in many stimulating activities.

When my sight began to deteriorate, my life drastically changed. I have macular degeneration in one eye and glaucoma in the other one. I couldn't see much at all, and I was utterly destroyed. I found the loss excruciating, and I cried and withdrew for a number of months. As my sight continued to fade, I couldn't read and could no longer see faces. I realized my eyesight was going and couldn't be reversed. It's now been at least eight years since I've seen my own face in the mirror. I've actually forgotten what I look like. I'm considered legally blind.

The loss of my sight affected everything I do, everything that had been important to me. I had been active as a handwriting analyst and had recently worked on a forgery case. I had also started to write a book. I had to give up driving, and that loss of independence quickly changed my life.

I've also developed some physical limitations. I can't raise my arms to do simple things because of pain I have in both shoulders. One of my shoulders has a torn rotator cuff, and the pain in the other shoulder is from a break that never healed right. One major frustration has been that I can't comb my hair. I have a dozen hats I can wear to cover my head unless someone is around to comb my hair for me.

I found I had the most difficulty learning how to walk with a white cane. From the very first, I found it pure agony, both emotionally and physically. I felt insecure and embarrassed. It was humiliating for me to think that people looked at me and most probably thought, "Look at that poor, blind old lady." I felt like a loser with a white cane. I almost completely lost perspective on myself.

Another issue I had to address is that I had no family living nearby, and although I was very apprehensive about giving up a place where I enjoyed living, I decided to move across the country to be close to one of my daughters. I settled into an apartment there in an active senior residence where older people live independently.

Shortly after that move I discovered an extraordinary center for the blind and visually handicapped very near where I lived. I decided to explore what it had to offer, and it's changed my life. I signed up to work with a mobility instructor who taught me how to use my cane with greater self-assurance. The kindness and skill of her instruction gave me a new feeling of security. I was gradually able to let go of that painful feeling of humiliation and regain my confidence.

What I learned helped me become far more competent. I suspect that I presented myself differently to the world when I felt self-confident, because people started to greet me on the street. It began with hellos and sometimes grew into conversations and new relationships. I began going out on the street, to the store, and to the local senior center. Little by little I began to build a new life.

I'm able to walk to the senior center from where I live. I can't cross streets without help, but the senior center is on the side of the street I live on. I take a class there from a totally blind woman who teaches tap dancing. I leave my cane at the door, the teacher takes my hand, and I dance with the rest of the group. I get hugs and kind words from so many in that group.

How do I spend my days? I still miss reading a newspaper, and I also miss my old habit of doing the daily crossword puzzle. But I have a lot of books on CD, and I listen and learn every day. I listen to the radio and to the news on television. I think about what I hear. I get very angry at injustice and hunger in so many parts of the world and in the United States too. I wish I could be more politically active. I feel strongly about the need for change in this country in so many areas. We have to improve our educational system, and it's appalling that we have hungry children in this country. I have an active interest in the world around me.

I recently went with a group from our senior community center to sing Christmas carols at a convalescent home. We all wore Santa hats and spent a few weeks making craft gifts to bring to the home. Everyone I saw at the center couldn't do things independently. Each person had a wheelchair and an attendant. Many things touch me deeply these days, and I cried after that experience. What a life lesson for me. I left there knowing how fortunate I am to have lost only my sight. I can still walk to the store down the street, hear audiobooks, and do all kinds of things. It was an enormous lesson in gratitude. I don't think I'll get frustrated in the future about what I'm personally lacking.

I want to tell you about my wonderful computer. Everything can be magnified, and my computer has a program that actually reads to me. I push two little buttons, and my computer begins talking. The center for the blind and visually handicapped that helped me when I first came here sponsored me for a state-supported program that sends someone to my home to teach me computer skills. A very nice man came once a week for several months and taught me so many useful things. It opened up my life. I have more computer skills now than I ever imagined I could acquire with good eyesight.

After a while I arranged for the wife of my computer teacher to come once a week to read to me. They've enriched my life enormously. These are people I never would have met if I had been sighted. Now they've become two of my closest friends. Friendship works two ways, and they tell me in different ways that our having developed a deep friendship matters as much to them as it does to me.

Losing my sight was terrible at first, but it also gave me the opportunity to learn firsthand that people with disabilities can do incredible things. I feel blessed in ways I never would have if I hadn't lost my sight. It may seem strange to hear me say that, but it's really true. I have fun and feel alive. So many wonderful things continue to happen in my life. I have a sharp mind, because I keep using it. I'm writing and talking with people. I refuse to isolate myself from the world. I'm open to new friendships and the commitment that takes. These rewards have enriched my days. At ninety I'm incredibly independent and it's a good time in my life.

I've come to realize that I used to miss many things when I was sighted. I've been enriched by blindness, and I truly, truly mean that. I feel touched, deeply touched, about things and people I would never have known had I not lost my sight, and I empathize more deeply with what's going on in their lives. I don't think I would have experienced these connections and emotions had I remained sighted. My life has been enriched in ways I never could have predicted.

> *Although the world is very full of suffering, it is also full of overcoming it.* —HELEN KELLER

Betty's story is not just about learning to survive after becoming debilitated, but also finding the motivation to thrive and enjoy new experiences in spite of her blindness. She has a strong voice, deep sincerity, and offers wise words. Certainly, not only *other* people are challenged by unexpected, unplanned changes in eyesight, hearing loss, diminishing general health, and limited mobility. We're all as vulnerable as Betty, whether we're young, in midlife, or in the later years of our lives.

In most situations, I've heard about family members who are exhausted from going back and forth across the country, working out a schedule with their siblings, and making daily phone calls to check in with the parent. Many situations aren't resolved as easily as Betty's was when she herself made the decision to move. She has been able to maintain and regain some measure of independence because of her move into an independent apartment in a senior living complex. With some measure of comfort, she has been able to adapt because of help from her daughter and services available in her new community.

I, and so many others, have often repeated that familiar but wise statement, "It isn't just what happens to you; it's how you deal with it." At any time, each of us might be challenged to cope with painful, difficult, and confusing experiences. Whether the event precipitating the need for a major living adjustment is an acute or chronic health change, loss of job and income, a death in the family, or some other dramatic event, we might do well to learn from Betty's story. Simply put, good can come out of unfortunate experiences. Learning and wisdom can grow out of unexpected situations. Life offers no shortage of opportunities to learn, to grow, to laugh again, and to enjoy new people and activities.

1. How have you handled major changes in your life or the life of someone in your care? Who or what has given you support and confidence to adjust to the losses and seek a path of recovery and healing? Does reading Betty's story give you motivation, inspiration, and hope?

2. Betty herself made the decision to move near her daughter, and it seems her daughter was also comfortable with the move. How have you or others you know dealt with the need for an adult child and parent to live close to one another? For a child and parent to reach a mutually comfortable living arrangement, what might be some elements of a helpful conversation?

CAROL
THIS ISN'T GOING TO SPOIL MY DAY

Enjoy life now; it has an expiration date!

—PRESIDENT HARRY TRUMAN

CAROL AT AGE SEVENTY WAS ACTIVE AND BUSY, LOVING AND fiercely opinionated. Her amazing life ended on a spring morning as a magnificent sunrise appeared. Along the way, her dynamic spirit and generous soul touched and inspired friends, family members, her condo community, and countless others. Carol was above all a devoted friend but also a champion of equal rights, a lover of the arts and education, a staunch opponent of anything remotely resembling ageism, and the incredible leader of her family. Her family felt loved and supported by their mother, mother-in-law, and grandmother.

Her friends will tell you that they've never known anyone so full of enthusiasm and determination. "She lived her life out loud," one friend told me. Carol showed us how to live and love, and encouraged us to laugh and celebrate life. She had a positive and profound effect on all who knew her. Those who loved her have said she will be missed immeasurably. She will always be with us, and for that we are incredibly grateful. As for me personally, our visits are vividly alive in my mind, and Carol's life-affirming attitude continues to be my inspiration to live each day fully.

She was in her freshman year at the age of sixteen at Cornell University when she met Peter, the love of her life, who became her husband and partner. When I met her, she had been living alone for fourteen years since his death.

When Carol and I had our conversation I had expected we would begin talking about her recent diagnosis of liver cancer, how she was handling it all, and what she was thinking about. But that wasn't Carol's way. Her life was filled with family and friends and stories of how their lives touched each other. That's what was on her mind.

If I could leave a legacy, what I'd like is for people to give one another words of appreciation now, both for the sake of the one expressing gratitude and for the person receiving the appreciation. Too often those words of praise or gratitude are spoken after a person is dead. I have a handful of old friends we call our lunch bunch. When we're able to all get together, we do this for each other. The generosity and kindness in this sharing is really beautiful.

I'll share with you the story of how my granddaughter came to a family get-together with fifteen empty boxes from a Chinese take-out restaurant. On each box, she wrote the name of one person at the gathering. Then she told us we had to write something that we liked, loved, or enjoyed about the person labeled on the box. Everyone wrote fifteen notes and put one in each person's box. Then we read the notes left in our box. The point of all this was that we received a gift of words that let us know we're special. There were smiles all around. People need to tell each other those things often. In different ways I plan to do that for the rest of my days.

My life was going along well for me. I had recently had two cancerous growths removed from my face, and I was suffering from gas and indigestion a lot, but I really didn't think anything serious was wrong with me. I had a regular appointment with my doctor coming up shortly, and a few days before, I started to itch terribly. So I had both my itching and my digestion problems to discuss with the doctor. My itching had gotten so severe that during the night I scratched myself bloody. When I saw my doctor she said, "I'm scheduling you for a CT scan on Friday." When I went back to her to get a report on the test, I saw in her eyes a look that meant "This is trouble."

I had two tumors in my liver and one in a kidney. She sent me to a specialist who said, "You have a very rare disease: cancer of the bile duct. Only two in one hundred thousand people have it. There's really no treatment." I was shocked at the diagnosis and even more shocked when he said, "The itching was caused by the bile collecting in your liver." The statistics were grim. Fifty percent of people with this diagnosis die within six months; twenty-five percent live a year.

My reaction? I was angry. I felt cheated. I had planned on living at least another fifteen or maybe twenty years, and I loved my life. Now the end was predicted. I started thinking about whom I wanted to spend time with and who and what was really important to me. My three sons and their families were in my immediate thoughts. I needed to be with them as often as possible. I didn't want to stop doing the things I loved to do. I wanted to see my close friends, go out to eat, go to lectures, performances, and other events. So that's what I did. For over a month I actually felt exactly the same as always. I had drive and energy. My son told people who inquired about my health that I still made the Energizer Bunny look like a lazy bum. Resting apparently is for those with nothing better to do, or so I thought then.

Now it's been almost eight months since the diagnosis, and I've slowed a lot. I have scheduled a nurse to come often and check out how things are going for me. I'm able to stay in my condo, sleep in my own bed, and enjoy my surroundings, but I need to sleep every morning and again in the afternoon. I don't go out to lunch much anymore, but friends bring lunch over to my place so we can share some time together. I still go out to dinner some evenings if people can pick me up and I've rested. No more driving. My social contacts are very important, and I want to spend time with people I enjoy. Most days I now have the energy for only one social engagement.

The most important things in my life are my friendships and provocative discussion. I'm interested in politics and the government in my state and social movements. I want to keep getting out two to three hours a day for as long as I can. Those are the things that feed me, that are important, vital, for me. I had signed up several months ago to go to a two-day Nobel conference at a local college. This year the subject was on the brain and neuroscience, and I really wanted to go. A friend who also was registered picked me up. When I got tired during the lectures and workshops, I went in the lobby and laid down on a couch, put my ear plugs in and my eye mask on, and took a nap. You know what? As I've gotten older, and certainly now that I'm sick, I've become more free to be me. I don't even give a thought as to what people think. I do what I need to do. It's very freeing.

I don't want people treating me differently. I want to experience as much of my life as I can have or as much as I can handle. Yes, I'm more and more limited, but I'm going to live my way until I drop. People often tell me that I'm teaching them how to die. They tell me I'm an inspiration, and I'm glad for that, but the truth is I just don't want to give up what I love to do until I have to.

When my husband died of lung cancer, he spent the last few weeks of his life in bed. I know that's going to happen to me eventually. My liver is going to fill up with cancerous tumors, and nothing can be done to save my life at that point. Then I'll be confined to my bed, and I probably will have more help at that time, along with my regular nurse, whom I trust and enjoy. It's a comforting feeling to know she'll be there for me.

People have been saying to me, "I can't believe how you're handling this." I don't understand that. How else should I act? I love my life, I love my friends, and I want to keep living until I'm not here anymore. People have been writing me e-mails and sharing their thoughts and memories about me. So many have told me in person or in writing how much having a relationship with me has meant to them. I wish that people wouldn't wait until someone is dying to tell each other how much a friendship has meant. Maybe to say such things could be a ritual for a holiday or at a special get-together of family or friends. Why wait until someone is dying to say those things? This can be my mission—to help people understand how important it is to ritualize in a personal way, with friends and family, the sharing of such things.

I've come to a comfortable acceptance, and at this point I don't have anger or denial, but I do feel cheated. I'm not going to get the years of life that I thought I was going to have. I was able to let go of that loss fairly fast, though, because I started to focus on what I experience every day, the good stuff, on what my life offers me today, at this moment, now. Isn't that all there really is—this very moment that's happening now between us?

> *Friendship is the happiest and most fully human of all loves, the crown of life.* —C. S. LEWIS

Carol will be remembered by many for her open, loving, and sincere appreciation of each of her friendships. Even in her casual encounters, she offered the gift of herself. What many might consider small stuff were big things in Carol's daily life. She found endless ways of offering kind and supportive words to others, to acknowledge their worth. Not only did she focus on that in our conversation, but during the years I knew her, I had often witnessed her also offering a special word or two at the conclusion of an encounter, sending a brief e-mail or a handwritten thank-you note, or wrapping someone in a hug. Carol connected with others by reflecting their worth. The many people she touched will always remember her. That is a priceless gift. She was one of a kind.

1. How might Carol's example influence you? How might you let another person know how he or she has enriched your life?

2. What aspect of Carol's story could enrich your day or your experience with others?

BOB

I CAN STILL SING AND LAUGH

The responsibility is on me for my success, no matter what circumstances I face or what difficulties I have to overcome. —ANONYMOUS

I RECENTLY RELEARNED WHAT LIVING IN A NEIGHBORHOOD means. When I was growing up I knew by name all the families that lived on our city block, both sides of the street. My current home is in a large group of condominium dwellings. Since I moved here I've taken the time to meet some families in the area where I live, bringing new people into my life along with their stories of challenge and inspiration.

I decided to attend an annual meeting of the condominium residents, and that was where I met Bob. He's a smiling man who uses a wheelchair that he's able to manage well without help. His interactions with everyone include enthusiastic conversation. It didn't take me long to learn that he had some inspiring words for me and possibly for you too. He was eager to tell me his experiences and was glad that I would share our conversation with you.

My first wife passed away. I did remarry, but we separated because I had to stay here where all my family lives, and she felt strongly about being with her family in Virginia. We had an amicable divorce, because we both recognized the limitations of our circumstances. I wasn't looking for another marriage, but I met my bride, my current wife, at my church. We've been very happy together, and I'm so thankful I have her in my life. She's been with me through everything I face now.

A drastic accident I had at work thirty years ago changed everything. My job driving a forklift was tough. One hot, dry day there was unexpected water on the road. I was driving the lift and lost control. I swerved and missed the guys standing on the road, but I hit a pole, and my forklift turned over. My neck was broken, and the forklift landed on top of me. When I was coming out of the anesthesia, I heard the doctor tell my wife that I'd be completely paralyzed. I was left with no voice and couldn't talk. I know I was crying. My wife and I quickly learned how to communicate: one blink was a yes and two blinks were a no.

My vocal cords were swollen so badly that no sound would come out. When I finally could make sounds, they weren't words, so no one could understand what I was trying to say. I could barely swallow food; and my hands didn't work, so I couldn't write. I had to communicate the best I could with my eyes and whatever facial expressions I could control. I could move my lips, so I could smile. I had many months of vocal therapy. It's amazing that I can talk so well now and even more amazing that I can sing.

I was in hospital care for almost eleven months. I remember the doctors told my wife that if I lived, I wouldn't ever walk, probably would not be able to talk, and most likely would not be able to use my arms or hands. After the hospital I went through many more months of physical therapy to get as much body movement back as I could. Saying my first words was so amazing. I remember when I could say them and my wife could understand what I had just said. She had tears in her eyes when I said, "I love you."

A critical factor in my recovery is that I believed I could heal, maybe not completely, but enough to live in this world. In spite of the doctors' predictions, I had courage, determination, an independent spirit, and strong religious beliefs. I had to work to heal, not to be angry, and to never give up.

Throughout my life I've dealt with and learned from emotional and physical crises. As a kid I saw that the more argumentative and bitter you are, the fewer friends you have or the more likely you have the wrong type of friends who drag you down. I learned that if I complained, the faster people would run away from me, so I pushed the anger, frustration, and fear away with prayer. I remembered how my grandfather and my mother both dealt with major health issues. In spite of the many challenges I was facing, I kept my focus on keeping people around me, and I always reminded myself of the good things in my life.

I'm in a wheelchair, my body looks normal, but it doesn't work. My arms don't function right, and my hands don't either. This wheelchair is my legs. It has become my buddy, my best friend. If it weren't for my chair, I couldn't be out and about doing my thing. If I didn't have it, I'd have to rely on somebody for everything. The key to dealing with a wheelchair is that you have to accept the reality of your situation. If you fight it and reject it, your independence will go right out the door. Your mindset is in your control.

Sure, I still have major pain, and I need to take painkillers. As we sit here I could be crying real easily. From my hips down, my body screams loudly. But I want people to know me and encounter me, not my disabilities and the pain I live with. It's my job to help the people with me adopt a positive, life-affirming attitude. I want to see a smile on the face of those I'm with. Maybe when they see my smile, they're thinking, "What does he have or know about life that I don't?" I want people to like what they see in me.

I continue to struggle with dressing, eating, and some regular activities. But I've got a comfortable home and a wonderfully supportive wife. I get to spend time with my grandkids, and my mind works really well. I love working in my garden, although I can't tell you how many times I've fallen out of my wheelchair and crawled back into it. I'm excited about living. Some people say to me, "I feel really bad for you," and I tell them there is no need to feel that way. I don't want anyone I encounter to leave me saying or thinking, "Poor Bob."

A lot of people have told me that how I deal with my stuff has changed their attitude toward their own inability to function, discomfort and other problems with their bodies, sadness, a whole range of stuff they're dealing with. I believe my example helps them take charge and respond in a more positive way. I know that my attitude is of major importance in my life. It's a whole lot better to live this way. It's a choice. I didn't want to choose the "woe is me" role. I want to help others. It's important to me. I'll do anything I can to get people to take on a different attitude, to put a smile on their face.

Just the other day a guy I met asked me if I ever complain. I told him that's it okay to complain. I have my moments. But when I'm done with my complaining session, I've emptied it out, and now I'm done. Complaining over and over puts off a lot of people. It's like a bad sore, and if you keep scratching it, it can't heal. Being positive is a behavior you have to remember and practice every day.

I now have an activity that I created with a couple of guys who play the guitar. We call our group Our Melody Moments. We do three-part harmony, and we go to nursing homes and sing and entertain with jokes. I'm in my fifties, and the other two guys are about ten years older. I'm the only one of our group who's disabled, so the other two guys set up the sound equipment and whatever we need. Someone donated a van to us, so we pack it up and away we go. The farthest engagement we accept is a couple of hours away. We just have fun, and everyone else around us does too. Some groups pay us a hundred dollars, and that covers our gas. Others can't pay us, but we love to do our gigs.

We bring folks back to their old memories through music and song. Some people at these nursing homes clap their hands or stomp their feet with the rhythm, and some even get up and dance. I'm so happy that I can talk, but even more grateful that I can sing. When I go to the nursing homes and other places the guys and I perform, it's really fun, and the audiences are great. I get smiles and hugs, and we stay after we perform and talk with many in the audience. That's a joy for my two buddies and me.

I was recently living in a nursing home temporarily for recovery, and I learned how easily people can be depressed. So often if you need help, you need to wait and wait, and it's difficult and can be depressing for many folks. I remember I had to wait to get the help I needed to go to the bathroom or to get out of bed, because I didn't have the strength to do that myself. Although I'm only in my fifties, I learned what it is like for people who are aging and dependent. I worked on developing patience and found that made a big difference in my comfort.

I often have encounters with people who feel hopeless, depressed, and sorry for themselves. I believe that they keep reinforcing that. I want to help them with my words, my music and singing, to let go of their depression and negativity and get on with their life, whatever it is for them at this moment. Depression is a harsh disability. I've felt it enter my life many times, but as soon as that happens, I counter that feeling. I say inwardly, "Get on with it; get this monkey off my back." Some people don't know how to let go. Many of us have times in our lives when we need help. We need to know that we can reach out and reach inward too. My way is music. I'm talking about the kind of music that puts me in touch with a positive, healing way to view the things in life that are most important.

My most inspiring message comes when I'm singing at a nursing home. Lots of folks there have lost hope. A lot of times, though, I think they're saying, "Don't fix me, just listen to me." I want to help them find a peace inside themselves, and I believe I can help others if I just listen. If people know you're hearing them, really listening, that makes a big difference. I listen to them and look at them and show that I care. I empathize and listen.

The way I handle the challenges and hardships I've faced is supported by my deep religious faith, my relationship with a supreme being. My religion is very important to me. It's a place where I can go, because for me, the Lord's spirit is in my heart. Without my religion, things would be far different for me. It's my gift beyond gifts. My faith guides me through my life. It helps me in how I live and gives me the hope that I can put a smile on the faces of others.

Relating to other people, even if religion as I define it isn't there in the other person, creates a bond. Others have their own way of dealing with their challenges. We're all connected. It's like you're in a pod, in the same pod, and you know there's no difference between the two of you. It's something you understand from within. My job here is to live each day to the best of my ability. I give to others through who I am and hope there's sunshine coming from my soul. It's as simple or as complicated as that.

> *To do the useful thing, to say the courageous thing, to contemplate the beautiful thing: that is enough for one man's life.* —T. S. ELIOT

Bob's determination and accomplishments, his healing and recovery from so many of his injuries, are amazing and inspiring. When he interacts with other people, he doesn't focus on what limited ability he has in his arms and other parts of his body. Bob lives in a way that puts the focus on the person he is. His disabilities will always be with him, but his pain, his sadness, or his personal concerns are not what he chooses to share. He's always available for others.

Bob's religion and his personal vision of a Higher Power are the core of his strength and his interactions with others. Each of us has our own particular religion or spiritual beliefs or support we count on. Bob has told me that his connection to a Higher Power has led him to his belief that all humans are connected to one another. He embraces that belief with love and a strong desire to serve others. I'm sure many who read his story will find that it helps them understand not only Bob but also themselves.

1. What portion of Bob's story offered a personal message for you? How might his story open a conversation for you with someone you're caring for, a class you're teaching, or a client you're supporting?

2. How does religion and spirituality relate to your life and work and the way you have faced a personal crisis?

3. In what way does an experience you've had shape your way of connecting with others either in your care or socially?

SULEIKA
I'M A WINNER

Heroes take journeys, confront dragons, and discover the treasure of their true selves. —CAROL PEARSON

SULEIKA WAS TWENTY-ONE YEARS OLD WHEN SHE BECAME ILL. Before her illness she was constantly doing things—finishing college, traveling to many countries. Her life at that time was an exciting adventure. Her travels and a job she had taken with a firm in Paris, and her future plans, were brought to a terrifying halt when a bad case of the flu left her with extreme exhaustion. Suleika's doctor suspected something more serious, and his persistence resulted in a diagnosis. This young woman in her early twenties would now have to deal with acute myeloid leukemia.

Back home in New York, her first round of chemotherapy lasted six weeks but offered no positive results. A second series followed; still no progress. Her doctors decided that a bone marrow transplant was a necessary next step. Her battle with cancer meant a repetitive scenario of getting in and out of various facilities. Her recovery was long, slow, often isolated, and a continuing challenge for her.

Suleika shared with me her memories and thoughts about the early days of treatment and her personal struggles, and her insights about finding a way to live with her new limitations. The medical world was making the appropriate medical decisions but offered no formula for dealing with the isolation and emotional distress of her treatment.

As I prepared for a bone marrow transplant, I discovered that my personal challenge might not be physical. The doctors would handle that, drawing on the remarkable advances in cancer treatment over the past few decades. But there is no magic pill to cure the emotional distress of a long illness. I quickly realized that my challenge was enduring the boredom, despair, and isolation of being sick and confined to a bed for an indeterminate length of time. I've since discovered it was up to me to deal with that challenge.

Facing my diagnosis of leukemia led me to see the world in a very different way. That first year was the most difficult of my life, but during those months I learned a tremendous amount about myself. I'm talking about both my limitations and my strengths. I was facing my mortality, and my understanding of what was really meaningful in life became very clear to me. At first I didn't want to learn these things. It felt unfair. So many things that had seemed so important to me, like my hair, which I spent twenty minutes fixing every day, suddenly weren't a priority anymore. I began to challenge myself and look inward to adjust to what was happening to me and find some meaning in it all.

When my first series of chemotherapy was over, my doctors did a biopsy and found that the treatment didn't work and my cancer had spread. It was then that I decided to move back into my childhood room at my parents' home. That was very difficult for me. I had worked hard in high school and college, and getting my job in Paris put me on my way to being an independent adult. Now I was back in my parents' home, and I was angry. I didn't really know who or what I was angry at, so I just bottled up those feelings. I didn't want to see my friends or my parents. I just wanted to be alone in my room. Everything I felt was negative.

I was this way for quite a while, depressed, isolated, and angry. It took me a while before I began to understand that I had to find a way to help myself. I don't know how it came to me that I should write about what I was experiencing. Writing is what I do, and it seemed a way for me to get out what was inside me, so I started. I wanted to confront myself on some of the issues I was facing. In the hope of helping the many others who share the struggle of a long and uncertain diagnosis or convalescence, I decided to tell my experience—the good and the bad, the deflating and the inspiring. I didn't write anything to do with my career. At that time, I didn't think I was ever going to have a career again.

I was beginning to feel guilty and realized that I wanted to be in touch with others again. I had gotten e-mails, phone calls, and letters from so many people, and I realized that I had ignored their concerns about me. I started with the thought that I'd write a message board online for my family and friends. But I soon discovered that many of them had passed on to others what I had written about my cancer, the treatments, and my honest feelings. During the first week my e-mails went out, even people I didn't know were writing to me and telling me they were going through similar things. Within a couple of weeks, much to my surprise, the *New York Times* contacted me. They asked if I'd write a weekly online column for them. It happened very quickly, and it was exciting but also a bit bewildering.

The response to my column was incredible. The personal stories that others have shared with me have given me an enormous amount of support and love from so many people I've never met. It made me aware of how generous and good and open-minded strangers can be. It's been encouraging to me, and I feel extremely fortunate. All the time I was in the cancer unit having my bone marrow transplant, I received many messages of encouragement and support. It was moving and meaningful for both my family and me.

Many e-mails were from people who were well, perfectly healthy. They showed me how many people appreciated their health and what they have. You know, I was quite young, had never really been sick, never broken a bone, and I had never stopped to think about my health. Now I really understand that it can be so unexpectedly taken away. I've learned that it's something I can't take for granted. All I have now is the present.

I wish I had understood that before I got sick. I now have learned to truly appreciate things, both big and small, very, very much. My life-threatening illness has given me a new and deep understanding of what *now* really means. I realized that I could help others as well as myself, and that they could sincerely and honestly share their deepest fears and their positive learning with me, giving me the emotional support and spiritual comfort I also need. So that's what I intend to continue doing.

Four years passed before I had an opportunity to talk with Suleika again. I learned that she had been told that she was in full recovery after her long months of early isolation and outpatient treatment.

I'm out of treatment and back living everyday life, and I'm thankful for that. I'm twenty-six now, and the life I had before my illness just isn't there anymore. It's gone. I write every day and post my thoughts on various social media sites, often about my transitions and how my cancer and recovery experience has left me with the challenge of figuring out where I fit in a world of women in their twenties. I share with others in this way, and many in return share reflections and comments about their personal experiences of transition. I'm not qualified to give them advice on how to live their lives, but often I share my personal thoughts in short pieces on social media sites. I've discovered I'll have many transitions to go through in healing and coming back into the world. I've learned a lot about myself and other people too from my experience in dealing with this illness.

I'm asked by different groups to tell my story of recovery, and I'm often invited to speak at hospitals, universities, and medical schools. I now have another subject I focus on as a former patient: I speak to doctors or those who will be doctors to help them understand that they are not just treating a disease, but that the patient in their care is also a person.

I'll tell you one personal example of some of my learning on that subject. When I was diagnosed and immediately began chemotherapy, I went on Google to look up the side effects of the chemo prescribed. I was shocked to learn that infertility was one. No one had talked to me about that. Here I was, only twenty-two years old, and I would never be able to have children. No one had thought that information might be important to me. The medical people had never asked how important that was to me. I raised my concerns and was told that they thought I didn't have time to take fertility-preservation treatments. I talked with my parents and my medical team about this issue. Together we decided I would wait three weeks for my next cancer treatment and do the preservation necessary for ten attempts for fertilization if I chose at sometime to start a family. What that taught me was that I needed an advocate who could look ahead with me and think about what might happen if I recovered and had a normal life. I needed to be more than a cancer patient seeking medical help. Communication between patients and doctors needs to be improved.

Now, in the hope of helping the many others who share the struggle of a long and uncertain convalescence, I've decided to continue sharing my experience—the good and the bad, the deflating and the inspiring. I've also taken on a mission to encourage the medical profession to find both the time and new ways of relating to patients and their personal thoughts, fears, and concerns as individual people. I hope my efforts will encourage patients and doctors to share conversations that are more personal and meaningful.

> *I am seeking, I am striving, I am in it with all my heart.* —VINCENT VAN GOGH

Four years after my original exchange with Suleika, I was visiting the city where Suleika now lives and was able to meet her for lunch and conversation. She now has an active and independent life. The subject of life transitions came up a number of times.

She's had an amazing recovery from the cancer. Her personal learning and deeper insights from handling a life-threatening illness have left her with interests and activities different in many ways from other people in their midtwenties. The battle between life and death has given her a mature view of her daily life and left her with priorities very different from those she had before her illness. Her insights and values are of someone much older, more seasoned. Looking youthful but having survived a difficult illness and arrived at a strange stage of maturity for a person in her twenties, her challenge is to explore how she fits into the world now.

As each of us deals with changes and challenges and the passing years, we're confronted with the question, who am I now that I'm not who I used to be? I've become aware that the answer to the question comes not from looking to the outside world, as many of us have done most of our lives, but from exploring the person inside ourselves and looking honestly at the person we've now become.

1. What have you learned from Suleika's story about dealing with unexpected illness or disabilities? Has your own or a loved one's illness and recovery given you a deeper understanding of yourself, your priorities, and how you want to spend your time and energy?

2. Has there been a time when you have been isolated because of your own illness, serving as a full-time family caregiver, losing a job, or any other experience? If so, how have you kept in touch with others during such a period, and what have been the benefits of these experiences?

3. How difficult has it been for you, or others you know, to realistically explore who you are now and to adjust to the ways

illness and recovery have changed your interests, abilities, and how a different pattern of life has evolved?

4. What is your experience or view of patient and doctor relationships? In what ways would you suggest the doctor-patient relationship could be changed or improved?

MARGE
POSITIVE WAYS TO LIVE

Even if the doctor does not give you a year, make one brave push and see what can be accomplished in a week. —ROBERT LOUIS STEVENSON

MARGE WAS IN HER EARLY FIFTIES WHEN WE TALKED. SHE HAD been active, busy, and content with life. Things were good for her and the family. Then everything changed with the diagnosis of a dormant condition that was now immediately life threatening. Marge and I talked about her coping, adjustment, and acceptance of the reality of her cancer now in its last stages.

This is one person's story, but millions have taken a similar journey through diagnosis, acceptance, adjustment, and continued living. Marge said she was comfortable talking about her personal experience. "Maybe something I've been through or facing now can comfort or inspire someone," she commented. "So what are we waiting for? Let's talk." And she began to tell me her story.

I was terribly upset and frightened eight years ago when I was diagnosed with breast cancer and had both breasts removed. I didn't think about dying at that time, because my treatment was working toward a cure, at least a remission. When I had that surgery I was very shaken, mostly because of what it means to a woman to go from being full breasted to having it all gone. Only one of my friends was willing to talk openly with me on a regular basis about my fears and sadness about the amputation of my breasts. Thankfully, she was able to lower the level of my anxiety, and I was gradually able to come back into the world of living. I had loved dancing and being active, and now I would have to dress differently and move differently. It was going to be a major adjustment. As I look back on it now, I was far more preoccupied with the loss of my breasts than with the possibility of dying soon. My breasts were an immediate loss, and I was going through the appropriate grieving.

Now, the cancer is back and has quickly spread. It will lead to my death. I'm in partnership with my dying now. My husband wants to plan, so we've scheduled some trips just for us and a few visits to family. We don't know if these trips will actually materialize, but when you're alive, you plan. Maybe it's just for tomorrow, but if you're living, you make plans. I know now that my life has prescribed limits, and my plans are colored with that reality.

This is a whole new way of thinking for me, but I'm actively aware of my dying in spite of knowing that I need to put my energy into living my life each day. My preparation for dying has become my personal way of easing toward an acceptance of my coming death. What I mean is that I need to believe that a tomorrow will come for me, although part of me knows that may not be so. You know, even if you're not dealing with a terminal illness, that's really true for us all.

People look at me differently now. I recently realized there's a look on their face that separates me from them. I just sort of feel it. I can't really define it, but I sense it when people change the subject to something light or trivial. I guess some people are afraid they're going to upset me or talk about things that will depress me. It's strange, but I often get the sense they think I'm supposed to make it easier for them. I do need to talk about my reality, though, so I often bring it up—not with everyone, of course, but with close friends and family.

As the months move on, I've become preoccupied with my dependence. I've wanted and have always welcomed emotional support, but I have great apprehension about accepting help with physical needs. That's something there's no way to plan for. For example, when I couldn't get to the toilet and needed help was a hard adjustment. How could I ever spend my life this way if I had to ask for help to do that? Well, that's my reality now, and I've come to understand that I'm going to have to learn to graciously accept that kind of help.

Each day I seem to resent my dependence less and even begin to appreciate that others are willing and actually happy to help me. I'm finally letting go of some of the terror I felt about dependency on others. I've come to peace with these fears, and I accept that my living now requires some help. How I deal with that is going to be my choice. If I need the help, I'll take it and be grateful for it.

I've come to a realistic acceptance of my life and my constantly changing limitations. My dying is an ever-present partner in my life now. But honestly, it doesn't depress me like you think it might. Yes, I'm going to die; everyone will eventually die. But my business today is my living. I don't want to think about dying all the time or talk about it endlessly. It's a disservice to the humanness in me. I'm living now, and that's what I'm going to do. Living is where it's at for me, one day at a time.

> *I lost my breasts, but I found my voice.* —ANONYMOUS

One of the difficult things Marge learned was how to accept help—to acknowledge that she needed it and to understand that others sincerely wanted to provide it. Learning how to accept help with personal things would probably present a challenge for most of us. Yet when we're no longer able to do some things without assistance, accidents can be avoided if we accept the care needed.

Coping with her illness in measured ways, talking about it with certain family members and friends, ignoring it at other times helps Marge to continue living even as her days are waning. Marge and her husband make plans for their future with the expectation she will live maybe one more day, maybe two, maybe more. Yet they both understand and accept that her body will eventually give out and those plans will not be realized.

Marge validates a truth that in our busy world we often ignore or forget: we all live one day at a time, whether we're aware of that reality or not. Here is a simple quote that Marge shared during our conversation. "I have come to understand that every day is something to cherish." That acknowledgment offers richness and an awareness to be embraced. It takes courage to push ourselves to places we have never been or understood before.

1. Have you had any experiences with others who are ill and aware that their death may be imminent? How have you handled such situations? Have you been open and willing to talk about death and dying when the subject comes up in conversation?

2. When have you heard of or been involved in an experience that has led you to a deeper understanding of time and appreciation of relationships and small things often overlooked in our busy lives?

3. What situation or event in your personal life has put you in a position to see time in a different way, possibly to understand more deeply the phrase "one day at a time"?

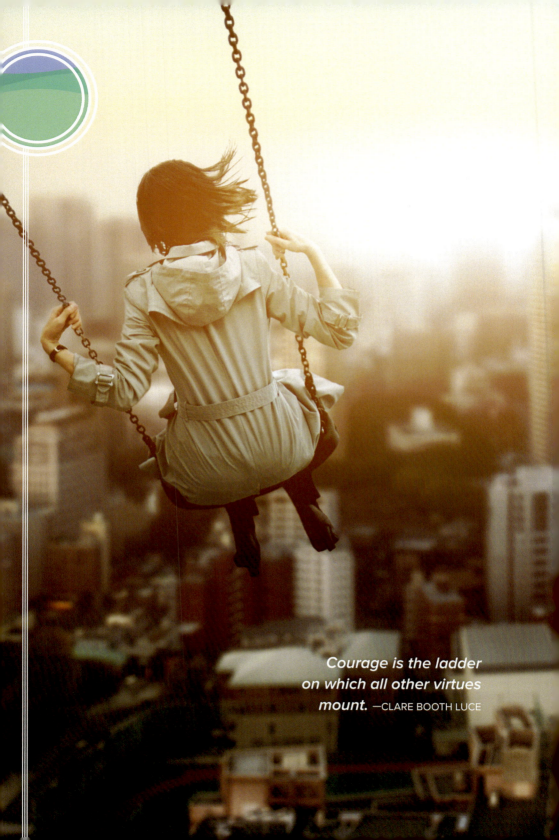

Courage is the ladder on which all other virtues mount. —CLARE BOOTH LUCE

RONA
MY SENSIBLE AND LIFE-AFFIRMING VIEW

AS I SAT NEXT TO RONA'S HOSPITAL BED, I WAS CERTAIN HER eighty-third birthday in four days wasn't going to be a celebration. Her eyes were closed, she seemed peaceful, and she was still breathing but very slowly. Her three grown children, who sat day and night by her side, knew that these were her final days. We sensed that when we spoke loving words to her, she heard them. A few days later she died with her family surrounding her and in no obvious pain.

Rona's memorial service turned out to be a celebration. It honored her as a good friend, a devoted mother, and a woman who lived every day of her life to the fullest. Indeed, she affirmed and appreciated each day after her diagnosis of breast cancer. In the last months of her life her health had deteriorated dramatically; yet with help she would dress, have either a lunch or a dinner with one of her children, a cousin, or a friend, and in appreciation of each day would radiate her life-affirming philosophy. When I had an opportunity to record a conversation with her several months earlier, she told me of the day she discovered a lump in her breast and immediately went to the doctor.

I drove myself to the clinic for the mammograms, ultrasound, and three biopsies. I remember wondering, what am I ever going to do if I hear that word *cancer*? It was my worst fear. So now the tests were over and my heart was pounding, and I called my kids and told them the bad news: it's cancer. I went home thinking, what now?

What came to me quite quickly were my mother's words. So many times I remember her saying, "If bad things happen in your life, how you face the problem and how you deal with it depends on your attitude." So I have cancer. How am I going to face it? What will my attitude be? I thought long and hard what my mother taught me. I'm the one who has the power to decide how I'm going to handle it.

For many days I thought about what I had learned twenty years ago, when my husband had his first heart attack. I lived in fear of him having another heart attack. What good did that do for me or for him? He ended up having three heart attacks and a triple bypass, and yet he lived twelve more years. I learned from that experience that living in fear, constant apprehension, and worry takes the daily pleasures out of living. I use that life lesson now, as I deal with my cancer.

I feel a connection to a Higher Power, something deeply spiritual. Some call it God, others refer to it as the Power or the Spirit, and many, like me, just call it dealing honestly and wisely with their constantly changing reality. I knew I needed support and help, not only from others; but I did ask my God to help me with the decisions I needed to make to get through whatever was ahead.

I don't ask, why me? All living beings are going to die at some time. I'm alive now, and I look at my life as a glass half full. I'm enjoying each moment. I even enjoy doing my laundry. I know that's a small thing, but I truly appreciate what I'm able to do. So many things that used to be so important don't really matter to me anymore. I always wanted things I couldn't afford. I now understand, those are material things that don't really matter. I used to dwell on what people did or said that hurt my feelings. Really, those things don't matter anymore to me either. They've become small things to me. The way I look at the world now has changed drastically. I'm going to try to find something good and meaningful in this experience. I look back, and I'm grateful for everything I've had and for the days ahead that I will have.

It all goes back to what my mother taught me. This cancer is something I can't change. I can only deal with how I handle it, the attitude I bring into each day. Now, every day I remember my mother's philosophy. It's not just what happens to you but how you choose to live with it.

> *People who are ill can produce moments of truth that heal mind and body and in the process reveal what really matters to us.* —JEAN SHINODA BOLEN

Rona's adult children asked me if at her memorial service I would read some of their mother's words from this conversation I recorded. That gave me an opportunity to share her philosophy with a full auditorium. At the reception following the service, many individuals told me their personal story about how as they spent time with Rona, helped her get dressed, assisted her in and out of their car or into a favorite restaurant, she listened to their stories and offered her wise and caring comments. They confirmed that her smile and her warmth reflected an attitude of appreciation for each day.

Rona has left an important gift for her family and all who knew her. How she dealt with the reality of breast cancer—not how she died, but how she lived—will remain her life-affirming legacy for all who read her words. Her story reminds me once again of the truth that we all can live only one day at a time. None of us knows if today will be our last day or whether we'll have many years ahead. Rona's life and her death gave us a gift, a reminder that our attitudes color and shape the texture of our days and those of others around us. Rona's life, including her last days, offer us a deeper understanding of what living is all about if we're open to embracing it.

1. **Have you ever gone through an illness or a health challenge that put you in a negative, hopeless frame of mind? If so, how did this affect your life, your family, your friends? Did you come to realize that a life-affirming attitude could make for happier days? If so, how did you come to that awareness, and how have you sustained this changed point of view? How might you help others by sharing Rona's story?**

2. **What has been your experience with friends, relatives, neighbors, or others who focus on the negative? Have you been able to help them adopt a more positive perspective?**

KENNETH
CONTINUED LEARNING AND COMFORT

> *It's not whether you get knocked down; it's whether you get back up.* —VINCE LOMBARDI

WHAT INSIGHTS AND WISDOM MIGHT WE GAIN FROM A TWENTY-eight-year-old man who has lived his whole life with Tourette syndrome, attention deficit hyperactivity, and fetal alcohol spectrum disorder? You might not expect to hear that this man, Kenneth, has written a book entitled *Makin' It*. It's his personal story, but the foreword points out that the book has been written for families, adults, and professionals who have family members in a treatment center or residential care facility.

Kenneth's truth was, and still is, that our care system provides needed physical care in a variety of safe housing situations. However, physical care and safe housing do not encourage disabled persons to understand and believe in themselves and build a measure of independence and confidence. Kenneth's personal experience, and his strongly stated opinion, is that professional helpers often miss out on some sense of the disabled person's own truth, one that could help each person build his or her self-confidence.

Every step of Kenneth's life has been a struggle and his days have been filled with many difficulties. Yet he is confident that what he has learned can help both those who need help and those who are the helpers. "When I was a kid and a young adult, a lot of people helped me grow up into the man I am now," Kenneth told me during our conversation in his small but cozy apartment.

Kenneth met me at the door with an enthusiastic greeting: "Hello. I want you to meet Amanda, my beautiful wife." The three of us settled down in their living room, and our conversation began.

My life has always been complicated. Figuring out what I could do, what I couldn't do, what was and wasn't possible for me was the big challenge of my growing up. Now I'm still learning every day, about myself and the world out there. I had to learn a lot about how to behave with a boss and others I worked with in my first job, a part-time one at a fast food place. I didn't understand the world of workers and employers. I lost that job. But I learned that I couldn't say yes to things I couldn't do, things that got me angry and stressed out because I was required to get them done faster than I could. But those are things about my life now. I want to begin our conversation telling you about when I was younger and share some things in my growing up years that were hard for me.

I don't remember exactly when I got the original diagnosis of Tourette syndrome, a brain disorder that often starts in childhood. It caused unexpected movements that I couldn't control, and I had no idea where they came from. Later, when my behavior was already totally unpredictable and unmanageable, and other behavior-related illnesses were diagnosed, I was told that I had fetal alcohol spectrum disorder, the result of my birth mother's drinking when she was pregnant with me. But my ADHD—attention deficit hyperactivity disorder, which causes hyperactive, obsessive, and compulsive behavior—came out of nowhere. The medical world was just beginning to understand some of the erratic behaviors and outbursts that come with such conditions.

My birth mother had a lot of mental health problems, and she gave me up when I was only a few months old, so I ended up in a foster home. I was about two years old when I started getting into everything. I'm sure everyone did his or her best, but I was difficult, the foster family had other children to take care of, and the decision was made that they couldn't keep me. I was told that they'd find me a "forever family." I was adopted when I was three and took the family name I now have.

When my mother had to have a heart transplant and my dad couldn't care for me full time, I was once more put in foster care. I remember I started hitting and kicking people at school. My behavior outbursts came often and were unpredictable. I couldn't stay in one place or sit still, and I was often wild and aggressive. As I got into my teens my reactions were out of control. My behavior frightened my father and often got him angry. He lost patience with me much of the time. I was just a kid and didn't understand that he had many of his own problems. It wasn't a good situation for me.

I was in and out of group homes and treatment centers and back with my mother only when she could care for me. It was often hard for the staff and others to understand me and know how to handle my behavior. I had to be supervised a lot, and much of the time my reactions were out of my control. Whatever my living situation, someone would quickly decide that I had to have what's called a PCA, a personal care attendant, with me all the time. I had hardly any freedom. I won't go into the details of how many treatment centers, residences, group homes, and foster homes I was in and out of, but my adopted family often couldn't keep me during the times when they were dealing with their health problems and other stresses in their lives.

Wherever I was, the staff and helpers assigned to me were always telling me that I couldn't do certain things because I had this disability or that. I wondered why they thought everyone with a certain diagnosis or disability was the same. That's when I first became aware that whatever home or facility I was living in, the staff judged me by what they were taught. My care was totally based on what they knew about certain limitations of that particular disability. I was always assured that they would take care of me, but what they didn't recognize or understand was how much I was capable of learning and doing. They didn't really care about getting to know the me inside my body. When I realized this, I got fed up with counselors, teachers, and other helpers who were in charge in the group homes.

I well remember some of my own efforts to look for the person inside my body that was so often out of control. One time when I was back living with my mom and dad, they heard about service dogs that were trained to help people learn some independence without supervision. My parents got me one of those wonderful helping dogs. His name was Limey, and he had been trained to take care of people who had the symptoms and behavior I had. He protected me, and it was wonderful to have that help and support as I slowly learned some independence and confidence.

After about a year and a half I saw that Limey had become the leader, the decision maker, and I followed. At first he had helped me feel more independent, but then I saw he was in charge of everything and that I had become totally dependent. Limey had helped me start to get out and gain some independence, but now my dog was making all the decisions, and I wasn't learning. I realized I had to start living without Limey, or I would never be able to be in control of what I could do independently in my life.

I began to learn about relationships with other kids and girls and what behaviors were right and wrong. These are things all kids need help, advice, and support with during their growing-up years. When I was teased or let people push me around, though, it took me a while to understand how to handle that. I had to live with anger, frustration, and stress. One thing I needed to understand was about girls and how to behave with them. I remember figuring out that one girl who was my closest friend for over a year wasn't the right girl for me. She was bossy and fussy and strict. She made all the rules and thought she owned me like a pet cat or a dog. I gave up that friendship, because I realized that she wasn't the right girlfriend for me.

I kept being moved in and out of one group home after another. I've learned how to handle lots of things in the group homes, camps, foster homes, and treatment centers I've been in. I want you to know that those experiences were important for me. They helped me get to where I am today. If I hadn't gone through some of the frustration, anger, and confusion at the places I've lived in, I don't think I would have made it out in the world. Even though the staff didn't help me feel that I could learn to be independent, I don't think I would have developed the amount of confidence I have now without their care of my physical problems, my body often getting out of control. I'm really thankful for that. But my body was only part of what was going on with me. I was having a really hard time trying to understand and control my teenage emotions and my coming into adulthood.

I remember the time I felt like I had a broken heart; actually it was like a broken soul. I was in the giving-up stage. I wasn't getting the understanding I needed. I was lucky to have family around me who understood that I was exhibiting physical reactions to my frustration, not only to my disabilities. I don't always get along with some of my family. But when I was in the worst of my frustration and uncontrollable behavior, they were there for me. What matters most to me is that my family never gave up on me. At that low point in my life, they were there for me. I needed a lot of love, caring, and patience. I was blessed to have my family.

How am I doing now? The problems of having some unexpected outbursts are still around, but I've learned that I'm resilient. I have to watch out because I too easily get to the point of overstressing, and my uncontrollable actions come back quickly. Having my wife here to be my support makes all the difference for me and for her too.

My mom and some others in my family didn't want us to get married, but finally they agreed. Living with my wife gives me a sense of comfort. We're here for each other, and I'm not lonely. When either of us is stressed or feeling down, we can talk or cuddle. Sometimes we don't get along, but mostly we share our lives. We understand each other's limitations and needs.

My dear wife and I have two beautiful cats. I have a job. I work at a local restaurant part time. I can walk there, because it's in this neighborhood, just a couple of blocks away. I do maintenance, like cleaning tables and taking the dishes to the kitchen. I have a job trainer who's working with me to teach me some other skills so I can get a better job. My life is good.

If you tell my story to others, maybe they can understand that people can learn and lead a good life even with the challenges and limitations some of us have to deal with. It's very important to me that I can help other people. My message for others is, don't run away from your problems. Push through them. What I want to say to those who provide care in treatment centers and foster homes is that as you give us the care and protection we need, leave space for each of us to grow into who we can be.

> **Faith is taking the first step, even when you don't see the whole staircase.** —MARTIN LUTHER KING JR.

I learned from Kenneth's experience that people often overlook the abilities of a living, functioning, thinking, feeling human being inside a body with unpredictable physical reactions. As for his mind, his thoughts, and his individuality, I learned a good deal in a ninety-minute visit with him.

I'm glad that physical care was and continues to be available for him if needed. Kenneth's adoptive parents give him love and support and have been with him through his many ups and downs. Unfortunately, Kenneth's awareness that he has intelligence, sensitivity, and a range of human emotions and reactions wasn't a concern or a priority for most caregivers who were trained to deal with the physical aspects of his disorders. Some well-trained professionals, including social workers and therapists, may never have gotten to know the person that I spent only a brief time visiting.

We live in a world of medical specialization and professionals, with specialists for every disease, disorder, and organ. Kenneth showed me that Tourette syndrome, ADHD, and other brain and mental illness diagnoses are dealt with the same way. Specialists focus on a particular disease or disorder. Kenneth, however, wanted me and others to recognize and respect that inside his body was a person with emotional, psychological, and social needs too. People who are deaf, blind, not able to walk, or possibly not able to talk may have thoughts, ideas, and desires. Our challenge, whatever intimate or casual relationship we have with someone, is to recognize each person's human complexity, not just the diagnosis or disability.

1. In your personal life or work, when have you discovered and come to know the person inside a patient or disabled person who had not previously been encouraged to emerge? What did you learn from this experience?

2. What has been your personal experience with the medical world? Do you have a doctor who treats you like a whole person or one who focuses only on the particular symptoms that prompted your appointment? Do you think specialization of medical care leads to depersonalization? If so, what do you see as the implications and possible results of this?

3. What changes in the medical world or the profession of caregiving are you aware of that have been modified recently to consider the person inside the body receiving medical treatment?

SUSIE
SURROUNDED BY LOVE

There are reasons to live everywhere you look, if only you have eyes to see them. —CHRIS HEWITT

IN THE EARLY 1960S NEWLYWED SUSIE AND HER HUSBAND CAME to Minnesota from the East Coast with no idea where they would finally settle down. The couple was determined to start an innovative community school, and the Minneapolis area looked promising. Many kids were dropping out of the public school system. Susie and her husband had ambitious plans to create an independent school that would be open to various ages. They were committed to helping troubled children get off the streets and continue to learn. With a smile and a bit of a giggle, Susie admitted that she thought the place her husband chose in the Twin Cities seemed like the end of the earth to a girl from the East Coast, but she was willing to try it.

Conversations, Insights, and Inspiration

Within a month of their arrival, they were offered the free use of a small island on a large lake outside the city. That's where they went to live and set up the school. Many kids who were having trouble at home or in school quickly gravitated to this place of safety and learning. Susie and her husband picked up the new students in their small boat and took them across the lake to the island school, which would also become a temporary home and a place of learning for the students.

Years ago, when the state authorized charter schools, Susie and her husband gave up their school. They now own the island and have spent many happy times there with family and friends. Yet going back and forth on their boat has gotten hard for both of them. They've recently had some serious conversations about selling the island. Taking care of two residences, one home accessible only by boat, isn't easy.

When Susie and I had our conversation, her life had been enriched by fifty years of marriage, the birth of her children, establishing and growing their school, and living on their beloved island. We sat comfortably in the spacious living room of the condo Susie and her husband now call home. Their island, directly across the lake, is visible from the large picture window. Susie wanted to talk more about their island with me, so that's where our conversation began.

Our island has been one of my main joys in life. I've really loved it more than any place I have ever lived. When I'm there, I'm totally at peace. I'm feeling teary thinking about the sweetness of those early days. Yet I realize now that as much as I hate to give it up, we're going to have to make realistic decisions. Life these past months has been relatively easy here in the condo in the city. It has allowed us to see how difficult the island is to manage at this time in our lives.

A little over a year ago I was diagnosed with endometrial cancer and underwent a complete hysterectomy. My operation was nasty, invasive, and much more serious than anticipated. The cancer had spread, and the surgery was considerably more extensive than the ordinary hysterectomy. I was told that my prognosis was five years to live and maybe not that long. When I heard those words and looked at my prospects, I cried a lot and thought about how I've always been a person who really treasures every day. Now I'm facing the hard reality of a limited life span and I'm aware that every day could be my last.

The reason I accepted your invitation to share my story with you is that I want to be an inspiration to others who might be facing personal challenges. I'm looking back on it now and remembering that after every chemotherapy session, I went through a period of being tired, feeling sick, not having an appetite, and getting exhausted just from knitting. I slept a lot, waiting for pain medications to kick in. I remember having little control over what happened to my body, yet I believed that everything would eventually be fine, even when things were tough. I was honest with everyone when I felt sick from the chemo or tired or weak, but I always tried to end a visit or a conversation with a hopeful attitude or a positive thought. Doing that actually made the whole experience easier for me.

I've had this positive, life-affirming attitude for as long as I can remember. I watched my mother deteriorate with cancer in her bones and liver, and she was very, very sick. When people came to visit, and in spite of how devastatingly ill she was, she would always have a smile on her face to welcome visitors. She'd ask them to tell her what they were doing and how things were going with them. Her conversations always focused on living, not her dying. Her way has become my way.

Lots of friends sat with me during my chemotherapy sessions. One friend who came to visit during those times always made me laugh. She knew what to say to bring me to laughter, and I can tell you honestly that it made me feel great. Being able to laugh in that situation really helped me experience the chemo treatments with a different attitude. People often comment that I laugh and smile a lot. My mother smiled all the time, and my kids have learned it from me. I don't ever want to stop smiling or laughing.

After each chemo session, I was confident that each day I would be better and that in less than a week everything would probably be back to normal until the next chemo session. Holding on to that view was my way of dealing with the negative side of it all. I don't want you to think this has been an easy, carefree journey, but dwelling on the negative doesn't help anything. I had to begin making the effort to come back into the world, but I needed to get used to baby steps. Our living room here in the condo faces south, and often it's warm enough that I feel like I'm in Mexico. I would often sit on the sofa, look out the window, and pretend I was at the beach.

I'm a very independent, self-sufficient person, and I've never been good at accepting help from others. I'm an "I'll do it myself" person. In this new situation, I began to see that I couldn't do this recovery thing alone. It was an important learning. To admit to myself that there were many things that I absolutely couldn't do now wasn't easy. I began to see that I needed practical help for meals, personal care, and other things too. Slowly I was able to learn how to accept help and how to recognize when it was necessary. I worked hard to change my thinking.

I formulated a rehabilitation plan that included handing some responsibilities over to others. I want to encourage those who resist accepting help to understand that it's both possible and necessary. Understanding the mutuality involved with accepting my dependence was another important learning for me. I began to see that others were happy to help, really happy to be asked to do things for me. I've always been the one to do things for others, so it took a very dedicated effort to turn that around. I didn't know anything about asking for help before this experience. Somehow, I was able to begin, and I was surprised when many were so willing.

I remember looking in the mirror one day to discover that I had forgotten what I look like with hair. I had a shiny, bald head with a few little wispy, white pieces of hair. It was still falling out, even though the chemo sessions were now finished. One day I pulled a bandana out of a drawer and tied it around my head. I really liked the way it looked. My seven-year-old granddaughter and I talked some about cancer, my surgery, and chemo drugs. For a youngster, she has a pretty good concept of what is happening to me. We talked about my lack of hair. During the few days that my daughter and granddaughter were staying here with me, we went together to a store that sold wonderful hats. My granddaughter loves hats, so she thought that I was really lucky to get to wear them.

One day I decided I had enough energy to go shopping for some birthday presents for friends. When I went into the store, I grabbed a cart just so I could lean on it. I came out of the store totally exhausted, which told me my energy wasn't going to come back automatically. I realized that I had to work on it. When I got home that day I made a schedule for going to the exercise room in our condo building. My daughter reminded me to stay hydrated and that mild exercise helped with the pain. She also suggested I try out the walking path behind our condo. I started to do those things and quickly realized that I was helping myself get stronger.

I decided to register for an American Cancer Society "Look Good, Feel Better" class. There were only three of us in my group. We tried on wigs and went from wigs to hats and scarves. They had a huge selection, and we learned many ways to wear the scarves. The leaders of our group were wonderful and patient. I actually had a good time. One woman in the group had been having a horrible day before she came to the class, but she left smiling.

During those early days of recovery I signed up for a cancer recovery course where we created a personal affirmation. Mine is "My positivity gives me power, strength, and energy." I plan to take those words through my whole life. We practiced taking a deep breath, smiling, and repeating it several times. I remember starting to see the light at the end of the tunnel.

Very early on I also connected with an Internet service called CaringBridge. I'd write something every day, or my daughter would write for me if I felt I couldn't. It's an amazing communication vehicle, and I felt like I was connecting with friends, family, and even people I hadn't known before. I was part of others' lives, and even new people began becoming part of mine. Writing about my recovery experiences was not only giving me support, but I found I was also inspiring others.

The day of my last chemo had finally arrived. I still needed to do blood draws a few more times and see my doctor in a month, and after that have a CT scan to see how much, if any, cancer was left. A friend and I went out to lunch to celebrate the end of my chemo treatments. I'm so lucky to have good friends.

I remember the day that my concentration came back. I could put more than five pieces together in a puzzle in one sitting, and I was able to concentrate on what I was reading for more than ten minutes. What a wonderful day that was. To be relatively pain-free and wide awake was actually a surprise. I'm happy to say that my days then began to fill up with ordinary things. I was so thankful that I could cook our meals, do the laundry, go shopping, and still have the energy to do my weaving and knitting. "Back to normal" meant going out to dinner with friends on Wednesday night and volunteering at the children's hospital on Thursday.

This cancer recovery experience has shown me how hard it is to give up things, even the small things, that I love and enjoy doing. I'm so grateful to have my life back again. A little voice in the back of my head says, "Be present and enjoy every day." This experience left me feeling like there are many things I need to do. That's what put me on a new, slightly urgent campaign to get my life in order in every possible way. I really know for sure that life is too short to save things up for another time.

I remember the day I was notified of the results from my follow-up CT scan. I went to the doctor's office to get the report. It really wasn't the kind of thing I want to find out over the telephone. Thankfully, the news was good, and the chemotherapy had done the job. For the first time in the whole adventure, I knew that at least for now, the doctors and I had knocked out the cancer.

The wonderful people in my life made my journey about living instead of illness, about hope instead of despair. This chapter of my life has lasted for over a year now. The tumor marker is down to normal range, and I'm not too much the worse for wear, but I will continue to take baby steps and listen to my body. My birthday is coming up, and I realized awhile ago I knew that I needed to celebrate this year more than I need to be celebrated. I feel like I have a whole new lease on life. Who would have guessed that this birthday would open this new door to my life? Thank goodness for ordinary days. I love ordinary days! This is an amazing way to live. I no longer have a black and white life; now it's all in living color. Life begins at seventy!

I have a list a mile long of things for which I am grateful. The first and most important things are the love, support, strength, and hope that I have received from everyone. I am oddly grateful to my cancer for letting me realize many things about life and living I wasn't aware of before. Positive thoughts, love, support, and prayers nurture me, today and every day. I'll be giving that support to others and to my husband too. I'm going to light candles today to the Virgin of Guadalupe and to health, not just for me but for many other people we know who are dealing with illnesses.

I am going to keep loving my life no matter what comes along. I have no complaints. I'm thankful for all the love and support that has kept me going and made it possible for me to get through the challenges of these many days. I've learned that the healing journey takes patience and time and courage and hope. Here's to more wonderful days! I'm in a place of peace.

> ***And what are you going to do with your one beautiful life?*** —ANONYMOUS

Our culture teaches us, from early childhood on, to value our independence. Parents are thrilled when a young child says, "I can do that myself." Yet a person recovering from a major surgery or dealing with an injury or a frailty can benefit from another person's help. Learning to accept an offer of help comfortably requires setting aside either temporarily or permanently (if necessary) the impulse to do something outside the limits of safety or common sense. Susie's story illustrates how the help offered was needed and appreciated but also affirms the value of again being able to help others.

I've found that holding back on suggestions but listening patiently as the person expresses her fears and apprehensions, emptying out the negative, is the best way to begin. The person in care needs that opportunity before any help can be offered. I've often then said something like, "I hear you." From that point on I might pick one of their fears and offer my experience of coming to peace with a similar concern. We need to realize that some fears might become reality and that the usefulness of alternative solutions depends on the outcome of a diagnosis or a surgery.

Smiling all the time isn't my nature, but I've learned from Susie what a blessed tool smiling can be. Something happens inside me when the corners of my mouth turn up. One day I tried smiling at my own image in the bathroom mirror, and the upbeat feeling I got from my smile resulted in an optimistic attitude for the whole day. Smiling isn't magic, but it sure can be an ingredient in a good day.

Susie's upbringing and the example of her mother were vital elements in shaping her ability to see her glass half full. Many of us haven't had a role model who plants what we could call the seeds of optimism. Negative responses often come easily to me, but I have been learning to abandon that response and consciously adopt a more positive reaction. If we believe that developing such an attitude is possible, unlearning a tendency to immediately react negatively to difficulties may be a gift we can give ourselves. Learning a more positive and useful attitude and unlearning an immediately negative and defensive reaction is possible.

1. What have you learned from your experience (or possibly Susie's story) that can help you help others who face major changes in their lives?

2. When have you helped yourself or someone else realize that negativity and focusing on helplessness and hopelessness can't resolve a situation but may actually create additional problems? How have you coped with such reactions?

3. How might you help others change negative language or a negative attitude? How might you be able to encourage a focus on the positives, the blessing in every day of the life each of us has?

SUSAN
AN ATTITUDE OF REGENERATION

Keep your face to the sunshine and you cannot see the shadow. —HELEN KELLER

SUSAN HAS A SERIOUS DEGENERATIVE DISEASE CALLED corticobasal degeneration. I met her through her friend who lives in Texas but who often gets on an airplane to spend a few days with Susan. My friend wants Susan to know that the people in her life continue to enjoy her company and value her friendship. I made a phone call to Susan, introduced myself, and asked if I too could come over and visit.

Before I went to her home I did some research on corticobasal degeneration, a disease I hadn't heard of. It's a rare neurological disease associated with progressive brain degeneration. Only one in forty thousand people have been diagnosed with it. It leads to the loss of brain tissue in the cortex, or outer layer of the brain, especially the area in the upper front section of the brain. Clinical diagnosis is difficult, as symptoms are similar to those of other diseases, such as Parkinson's. Currently there are no known causes and no cure.

When I visited Susan we sat in her spacious living room. Her speech is extremely soft, so we sat close to each other as she shared her story.

I was diagnosed four years ago, and as of today my neurologist has given me a life expectancy of seven to ten years. The label on my illness is corticobasal degeneration. I prefer to call it regeneration, because that's the way I like to feel about it. I've developed patience, because I need to have plenty of it to deal with this disease. I know the prognosis. Eventually I'm going to have feeding tubes, and I also won't be able to talk or walk. There's no medication for these problems, nothing to slow it up and no cure. Still, I try to keep a balance between hopefulness and acceptance. I really don't always know how to do that, but I keep learning how to be on my own team. That's my challenge.

My brain is affected on the left side, and as a result my right hand doesn't do what I tell it to do. It doesn't work at all, so I can no longer write. It doesn't scratch my scalp right either. I'm sure you've noticed that my voice also doesn't work right. At this time my activities are somewhat limited. I fill my days with reading, and I belong to a book club. We have interesting discussions. I need exercise, so I walk every day. I take sleeping pills once in a while and arthritis medicine if I feel I need it.

It's vital for me to retain an upbeat and optimistic attitude, and sometimes I can do that more easily than others. Often when I wake up in the morning, for a moment it's like the old days, and I've forgotten about my limitations. Then for a few minutes I'm depressed. I do have some bad days and sad days. Those times come when something I could do yesterday I can't do today. Most probably I will never be able to do that thing or move that body part again. That's always a sad time for me. There are also times when I'm so weary that I want to just give up, go to sleep, and hide from the world. Yet somehow another part of me says, "Get up and live." I want to be a positive example to other people who are dealing with illness and disabilities, so I practice holding on to a measure of hope and optimism.

Before my illness, I was very active. I was a partner in a management group for several years. I always did volunteer work, too, at a home for single moms and their kids. I formed a mentoring program for them. It's a transition program to help them make the move out of the home, finish whatever training and schooling is necessary for the job the moms want to find, and avoid falling back into the situation that brought them to the home in the first place. Depression and lethargy are what they're left with, and they need a support system to keep them from falling back into destructive behaviors. Now I need that too. I'm thankful some of my friends are able to give me that.

I've also had many years of dealing with the challenges of my family situation. My daughter was chemically dependent, and my husband and I raised her two sons. She's in a women's shelter now with her son. I guess I've learned a lot about limitations and challenges, and I know how to offer support.

These days I have to put much of my energy into being a support for myself. I'm getting to the point of disability when some of my friends seem to be uncomfortable around me.

I think I'm a reminder of their aging, their slowing down, and their mortality. Some people aren't ready for that awareness. I wish they could understand that it's the same me inside this broken body.

One thing I'm having trouble coming to terms with is my increasing dependence. I'm not yet really very dependent except for a couple of small things. I can't get my bra hooked in back anymore, so I have to have my husband do that for me, and I hate that. I can't write checks; in reality I can hardly write at all. I'm having a hard time e-mailing messages too. As you can tell from the conversation we're having, I can't talk very well anymore. Many of my changes are similar to Lou Gehrig's disease (ALS), but in that illness the disintegration is quicker.

I knew I needed to build myself some support as I began living with my illness. I'm Catholic, and early on I went to my priest, and he encouraged me to develop a personal relationship with a Higher Power. I'm in a centering prayer group now. I have a personal prayer life, and I've learned that silence is my first language. It has become my way of digging deeper into myself. It's the way of getting underneath the face and the behavior that we all put out there in our culture. I've joined a small community for centering prayer and yoga. That has been my inspiration and my strong inner support. I meditate, and that's how I connect with my spirit inside. I believe there's a higher being inside each of us, and I've found something inside me that has become a personal partner to my religion.

As for my physical care, I expect at the end I'll need to be in a hospital. I'll also welcome hospice care. You might be surprised when I tell you that my disease has been a gift to me. I'm calm and more centered in my being, and I really know who I am. I've grown more comfortable in my own skin and feel ready to face my future.

> *I make the most of all that comes, and the least of all that goes.* —SARA TEASDALE

Almost a year after my conversation with Susan, I learned that she and her husband had moved to a retirement community that offers full care when needed. Her speech is greatly diminished, and her memory is unpredictable, yet she welcomes visitors with a smile. Our mutual friend told me that her confusion is intermittent, yet there's a peacefulness in her that has become part of her nature. She values what life she has left and is living as fully as she is able.

I've learned from Susan and others I've talked with over the years that inside each of us is a quiet place that we often ignore, neglect to nourish, and perhaps do not even discover because we put our time and energy into our busy lives. Of course, each of us has obligations, families, work, and responsibilities. Our outer lives are filled with doing. Yet, when illness, disability, and aging bodies slow our pace, whether temporarily or permanently, the still, quiet, deeper inner self can emerge. We can ignore it or embrace it. We may feel it is in our way, or we may discover it has given new meaning to our lives.

A person doesn't need to be facing a disabling disease to slow down. One gift of slowing down, though, can be the opportunity to know who we are on the inside, not just the outer image we've created. We can discover a deeper self at any age, any life stage, in any situation, if we consciously choose it. Susan's life may end soon, yet the deeper sense of being she has found within herself may offer a life lesson for all of us.

1. What does Susan's story say to you? Does the fact that she's slowly dying yet discovering an inner peace surprise

you? Have you witnessed or heard about others who have found peace in a difficult circumstance? If so, what have you learned from their peacefulness?

2. I've been told by two of Susan's friends that they and other friends and neighbors feel comfortable visiting her, although the few words she shares are barely understandable. What is there about visiting a person who is in touch with his or her inner self that eases the fear of death and dying? What experiences have you had with someone who has discovered such depth and peacefulness within?

BARRY
WINNING MY BATTLE

> *Every time you meet a situation, though you think at the time it is an impossibility, . . . once you have met it and lived through it, you find that forever after you are freer than you were before.* —ELEANOR ROOSEVELT

WINNING THE BATTLE AGAINST CANCER, OR ANY LIFE-threatening disease, may grant us not only a physical victory but also an unanticipated and inspiring source of spiritual deepening and profound insights. This story is one of millions about someone facing a life-threatening illness that not only brings struggles and pain, but also opens the mind and heart to a new understanding of life's priorities. Whatever disease or health challenge you or your loved one is facing now, or has dealt with in the past, this story may offer insights and inspiration.

We hear stories of people facing a dreaded illness, coming through it all, and returning to normal life. It's never exactly the same life they left behind. Barry's story is one of many about a recovery from a life-threatening illness. I'll let Barry introduce himself and tell his story of the challenge to survive and unexpected learning about himself that opened the door to life-changing priorities.

I'm fifty-six years old, married for over twenty years, and my son is eighteen. I've been passionately interested in theater since my mother took me to a children's play when I was around ten years old. I wanted to act and perform like those people on the stage. I was able to go to a theater school when I was young, study mime and acting, and start designing and directing plays. For many years I've been busy, productive, and creative. Eight months ago this chapter of my life drastically changed.

For several months, my doctor had attempted to relieve a terrible pain in one of my hips with various painkillers, exercises, and limitations of my physical activities. Nothing worked, and the pain became worse. Ultimately a bone biopsy identified the problem. It was late afternoon when the doctor called and told me to check in to the hospital at seven the next morning to begin chemotherapy treatments. The diagnosis was non-Hodgkin's lymphoma, stage 4.

I naively asked if I could wait a couple of months, so I could take care of my obligations in the work world. "Absolutely not," was my doctor's response. "Without immediate treatment, you'll be dead in two months." He continued to explain the disease, and I began to grasp the life-threatening seriousness. I was in shock and disbelief, and I felt like I was having a nightmare. My wife and I packed my suitcase as we struggled to understand a disease and a treatment we knew almost nothing about.

Many people might ask, why me? My question was, why now? I had contracts to direct challenging and interesting theatrical productions. The number of jobs promised a year of tight schedules and, at last, financial security. As for going into the hospital the very next morning, I realized I didn't have a choice. However, looking back, I understand I did have one very important choice. That choice was to fight to stay alive. I chose the path that offered that possibility and checked into the hospital at seven the next morning. My first chemotherapy treatment was two hours later. I was assigned a room at the hospital that became my home for the next five and a half months.

As I started to adjust to my new reality, I began to see that we are not in control of many things in our lives, even when we think we are. The only thing I could control was how I reacted to this new situation. I was a relatively young, healthy, active person, and now everything had changed. I didn't come to this realization gradually or have the option of choosing a convenient date to begin treatments. My train got derailed in one big swoop.

Very soon after I entered the hospital, the medical staff told me the chemotherapy treatments would be so intense that I had to be monitored constantly, day and night. I told my doctor that I was used to having a project to work on and I asked if I could make this cancer challenge my project, too, and somehow work along with the medical staff. I told him that I planned to ask a lot of questions. Doctors don't usually have this kind of a relationship with their patients, but I emphasized with a good deal of passion how important being actively involved was to me. Thankfully, my doctor understood what I was asking and was direct and clear in every explanation that followed. I wanted to learn in detail what was happening inside me so we could then take on the healing project together. I guess I was thinking of my cancer treatment like I think of my involvement in a theatrical production. Maybe I was a bit naïve, but I felt I needed to be an active participant in the fight against the cancer. It was kind of like getting a play ready for a performance. It would put me on the team to kill the cancer in my body.

I had conversations with my doctors every day about the specifics of my treatment. They took time to explain what they were checking and what they were doing to me and with me. Understanding those details made me feel a part of the army of doctors, nurses, and special consultants. We were all out to kill the cancer. Of course, I couldn't do anything except cooperate with those who were doing what the medical team decided was needed. I worked hard to keep my attitude positive and my conversation optimistic, and to hold on to my determination to beat this horrible disease. The hospital had its team, and I had mine. My wife, son, mother, and sister, along with many, many devoted family and friends, were there for me. I never underestimated the power of their positive healing thoughts, supportive actions, caring, and love.

Every day brought new challenges and difficulties in managing my physical reactions to the intense chemotherapy. The white blood cells that carried the cancer throughout my body were multiplying fast. The chemo drip lasted over twenty hours. I had nausea and diarrhea. I often wasn't able to drink or eat. I was weak and exhausted and at times ran a fever. I was confined to the hospital and in exhausting treatment for almost six months. Today, as we're having this conversation, I've been living back home for about eight weeks.

When the chemotherapy was over, I was given several follow-up tests to see if the cancer was still in my body. If it was, I was told I would have sessions of radiation. To my enormous relief and great joy, all results indicated that I was cancer-free. I was, and am, so very, very thankful and forever grateful to my wonderful doctors. I'm hopeful I can remain cancer-free and live for maybe thirty more years. Hey, I'd only be eighty-six, and these days many eighty-six-year-olds are living a good life.

I had so many friends all over the world who prayed for me to their God, the saints, or Buddha. Some wrote to tell me they did healing circles, chanted with groups of friends, or prayed for my recovery in their church or synagogue. I'm grateful to them all. There was strength in the spiritual mix. Their goal was the same, to see me well and active again. I was deeply moved by the depth of friendship. A friend made a pledge to her church in my name to be delivered if I recovered. She's taking me to her church this week to offer a generous donation to show her gratitude.

My medical team told me that being in recovery is a process that can take a minimum of a year before I'll be close to normal health and energy. Soon I'll be scheduled to go into a rehabilitation facility for a few weeks. I'm still weak, and my body is only about 60 percent working again. I'm still on many medications, because I'm extremely vulnerable to infection. At this point I'm learning how to deal with a slow process of recovery, accept it, and live with it. For almost six months my priority was fighting death. Now my number one goal is to get with the slow but honest pace of my recovery. The whole experience has left me physically, emotionally, and mentally in a different place. Those who visited me during my time in the hospital will see me looking very much like the person I used to be. My hair is growing back, and I've gained some of the thirty-five pounds I lost during treatment. But I'm not the same person in many ways. Looks can be deceiving.

People around me can't possibly conceive of what I've been

through, how little energy I have now, and how their expectation that I will be the person I was before the illness cannot be fulfilled. I understand where they're coming from. They want to resume the pattern of our previous relationship, yet my so-called old, normal life—being constantly overscheduled, always working, traveling, and planning the next theatrical production all at the same time—has changed. I see now that creating the same overly busy schedule will no longer serve me. For many weeks that busy life has been over, and I've spent a lot of time inside myself. My vision of how I'll live in the future and the choices I'll make has changed.

What I'm learning now is that I must set new priorities and respect and honor what my body is telling me. If I start feeling an overpowering exhaustion, I need to stop what I'm doing and tell whomever I'm with that I must sleep for a while. This is a total change. I can't do things at the pace I used to do them. I get that message every day, loud and clear.

My old life was tightly scheduled. I've been multitasking for years. I couldn't say no when an opportunity to direct another play came along. *No* wasn't in my vocabulary. I didn't turn anything down, and I didn't want to lose new contacts or disappoint others. In my early days in the hospital I began to look back on the events leading up to my diagnosis. Warning signals had flared up and manifested themselves in symptoms that I didn't give my attention. I had severe pain in my hip, bone aches, sleepless nights accompanied by night sweats, and weight loss. When I looked at my travel schedule, the rehearsals I had scheduled in different cities were often separated by only a sleepless night or a long train ride between cities. There were no real pauses or breaks, no safety net. I had lived that schedule for many years. I could see it only as I lay in a hospital bed. I won that battle, and now I will live a different life.

However, I'm not in the world I was in before the cancer. My brush with death has altered my priorities in life.

Yes, unlearning my old ways and the overly busy, overly committed part of me is going to be a real challenge. In today's world so many of us see great value in constantly staying busy and having the feeling of being productive. It's how we feel others judge us. But I'm here to tell you, and anyone who will listen, that people can grow and change from having an experience they didn't choose and hoped never to have in their life. I'm talking about positive learning coming out of a negative experience. I realize now that letting go of and unlearning the pattern of my adult work life is going to be a big challenge for me. A gift of my experience with cancer is that I'm discovering a new me inside.

I'm also continuing to learn to listen to my body's needs. My body has a voice, and I've learned to listen. Killing this terrible cancer has not only given me back my life but has also opened my eyes to a more balanced way of living. Cooking a good meal, taking a walk in the park, working in my garden, and doing simple things can be as important to me as the praise I get for doing what we all see as the big things, the visible accomplishments.

The world moves much faster than I do these days. Friends want to make plans for next week or farther ahead, and I just can't do that. I can only deal with the day I'm living now. I never know when the exhaustion will hit me. Lots of people around me want to label me "recovered," because I'm no longer in the hospital, but I'm not ready to overfill my calendar with work, social commitments, and every new project that comes along. It's easier for others to deal with the old me, but that person inside me has changed.

My new discovery is that there's a life after work. My plan

for the future will be about balance. I'm not only building up my health and my strength, but I'm also growing into a new me. I'm finding inner peace while just sitting in a garden, walking in the woods, or watching a squirrel break open a nut. I'm seeing my cancer as a gift that has helped me get a new perspective on my entire life.

> *Everyone has two lives. The second one begins when you realize you only have one.* —STEVEN SOTLOFF

I once read a comment by a doctor that people don't pay much attention to their health until they lose it. Dealing with a life-threatening disease can require full-time focus, and a new vision of life's priorities can emerge. Barry's decision to be an active and involved partner in his treatment, with the acceptance and cooperation from his doctor, was a unique approach that made possible his understanding of each of the difficult and painful steps along the way.

Barry's story, like so many others, confirms that an unexpected, uninvited health crisis gets our immediate attention and changes our priorities. I recall a conversation I had with a woman recovering from major surgery. She offered this life-affirming comment: "No one get's out of this world alive, but while I'm here, I'm determined to live to the fullest with whatever comes into my life." That's exactly what she did and what Barry's decision has been. Each of us can do the same. We don't necessarily have to face a life-threatening illness or debilitating injury to reassess our priorities and choose a more meaningful direction for our lives.

1. Have you, or someone in your life or experience, actively participated in the treatment and healing process? Do you believe the healing process can benefit from consciously taking on attitudes and actions of active participation? Why or why not? What might be the benefits of being a more active participant in treatment decisions?

2. What experiences have you had in your own life or with others in your personal or work life to change the priorities and the pace of living? How has that decision enriched your work or your personal life?

3. How does a person who regains his or her health hold on to such life lessons and not fall back into old patterns? How do you hold on to new insights and wisdom?

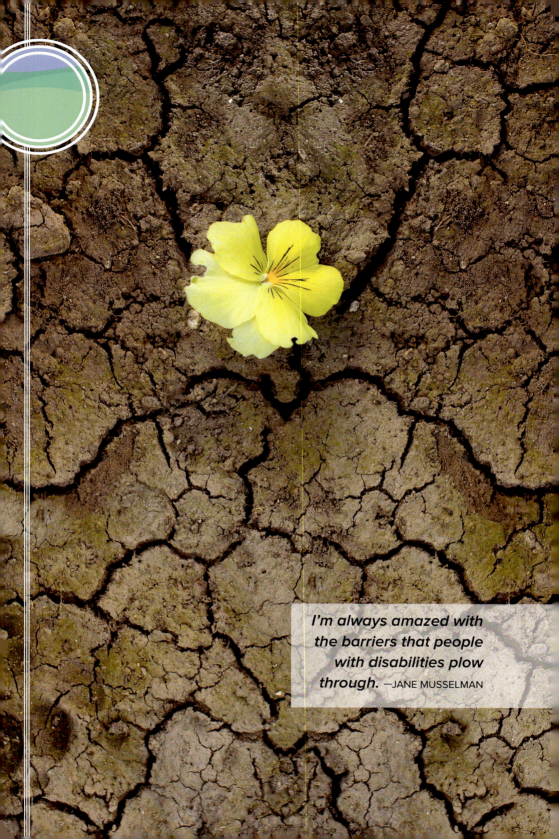

I'm always amazed with the barriers that people with disabilities plow through. —JANE MUSSELMAN

LASHA
LIFE'S SLOW RECOVERY

THE WEATHER WAS PERFECT. ICE ON THE ROAD HAD LONG SINCE melted on the narrow country road. Lasha's cousin was driving, and she was in the back seat of the car. Lasha had just nursed her baby, and she was reaching to readjust her seat belt when the car hit a stretch where the road had washed away. The car veered off the road and rolled over the embankment, flipping over as it went down the hill. Both Lasha and her fifteen-month-old daughter, Mika, were thrown out of the car. Her baby was killed, and Lasha was seriously injured. At the hospital, most of the medical staff quickly gave up on saving Lasha.

Although we rarely hear doctor stories like this, one doctor stayed with Lasha through the night. I don't know how often he might have administered whatever procedure saved her life, but when the new day dawned, there was a chance she might live. Months of medical care followed until finally she was able to ride in an ambulance to her mother's home to continue her recovery. During the months when the physical wounds were healing, her brain had its own pace for recovery. Lasha now continues to live the story she tells us here.

I'm thirty now, and the car accident was nine years ago. One of the things that happened to me was a very bad brain injury. I was in a coma for something like eight days and wasn't aware of how near death I actually was. I only learned that from people telling me the story two or three years after it all happened.

My fifteen-month-old daughter, Mika, died in that car accident. Even before I was told she had been killed, something inside me already knew. When I was in the coma my daughter had come to me in a vision. She talked in an adult voice and told me that I had to stay here, that there was a reason for me to live. She told me she was with her grandma and great-grandmother. She said that she had to be on that side of the stream and that I had to stay on this side. Because she came to me then, and still often does, it's easier for me to adjust to the reality of her death.

Some people may not believe Mika spoke to me, but her words gave me the strength to keep fighting and to get better. Of course, many days I still think about her and I feel very sad. I've come to understand that it was her time to go, but it wasn't mine, and what she told me gave me the strength to keep fighting and to get better. In spite of the continuing health challenges I've dealt with, I have confidence in myself and in my determination to handle my life.

As a result of my brain injury, I have had to learn how to remember. I had to relearn the alphabet, how to read again, how to spell, because I had forgotten everything I once knew. I was in every kind of therapy possible—speech, vision, physical, and whatever else they could offer me—and I was eager to accept the help. Every day I learned things that I knew before the accident but that my injured brain had forgotten. If I couldn't do things, I just accepted that I couldn't do them. Something in me knew it was a process, and I didn't feel the frustration many people expected I would. I believe recovery was easier for me because I accepted the pace my body and mind needed to recover. Nine years later I'm still relearning something every day. I'm still in a brain-injury support group, but I've come a long way.

Something my deceased daughter, Mika, told me was that I needed to stay here and take care of all the people and children I care about. I took that instruction very literally. One thing I knew for sure during my recovery was that I was going to include as many people in my life as I could. Before I was injured I had gone to school, gotten a certificate in child care, and worked in a preschool setting. When I was able to work again after the accident, I started doing foster care. At first I did that mostly on weekends or for short periods. I don't remember how long I did that—maybe three, five, even six years. I did that for several different families. I have always had a very comfortable bond with children, and my relationship with foster children continues as they grow up. I keep in touch with every one of them.

A number of years elapsed after my first conversation with Lasha. When I had an opportunity to talk with her again, I was reminded that we often ignore the fact that the healing process has a beginning but not necessarily an end. Both Lasha's story and her healing continue.

I remember when we had our first conversation, I told you that my daughter who died in the accident came to me in a vision in the hospital and told me it wasn't my time to go. So, I'm here, and I keep learning and healing and living my life to the fullest. I now have a husband and three young children, and I work as a masseuse. Before the accident, I always wanted to be an elementary school teacher and work with children's minds. After the accident, I became more interested in the body, and I trained as a masseuse. I also studied to be a healing touch instructor. I'm now certified to do infant massage. I work with children up to the age of five and instruct parents on how to work physically with their children. My massage work now includes young people of all ages, and also adults of various ages, some in their eighties.

I've had to deal with many emotional and psychological challenges these past years, and new challenges continue to confront me. I get frustrated when I want to do something that was once so easy, almost automatic for me. Reading is one important example. I don't recognize some words that I know were once familiar to me. It takes me a long time to read a page. When I took a class recently, I had to have the book in audio format, because the pace of my reading is so slow. Other people can read a whole chapter in the time it takes me to finish one page.

I've taken on new obligations, and I live at a different pace than I was able to handle right after the accident. I've forgotten how to handle many things at once, like I could before the accident. My old way of doing things is gone. I've found that when I have specific things in the house to do for the kids or my work, I get them done, but by the next morning I've totally forgotten what I did.

I've gone back to the therapist to get help in figuring out how to deal with these new challenges, and with her help

I've developed some different planning and organizing skills. I've had to learn a new system for dealing with my files and remembering what's in my piles, or I can't get everything straight. I have a new way of making lists, and I make them short, so I don't get overwhelmed and confused. I now have a folder for each day, and that's where I write down what I need to do at home or with the kids or for my work, or things I need to remember about my clients and appointments. I'm sure I once knew how to plan and handle these things, but I've had to learn them all again.

For many years I've been in a brain injury group that meets once a month. I see some people who give up trying to regain some of their competence. I'm not going to give up the fight. I have confidence in myself and in my determination to handle my life. Yes, I'm always going to have problems from the accident. Sometimes I can't really keep up with everything I plan for a day. I can't breathe well, so I always carry an inhaler. When I do too much physical activity or it's cold out, my breathing speeds up and my body aches all over. I'm used to that now, and both the symptoms and the solutions have become a permanent part of my life. Sometimes I get migraines and my vision becomes blurred. I've now learned to stop what I'm doing, go for a walk, rest for a while, and sometimes even take the remainder of the day off. I really have to watch out for exhaustion. I need about ten hours of sleep every night.

Much of my life today is about learning and compensating and compromising. That will also be my life in the future. I remember when we had our first conversation, I told you that my daughter who died in the accident came to me in a vision in the hospital and told me it wasn't my time to go. She's always with me. So, I'm here, and I'm going to keep learning and live my life to the fullest.

> *Life has got to be lived; that's all that there is to it.* —ELEANOR ROOSEVELT

Much of Lasha's recovery has been about putting in the time, effort, and commitment to relearn both simple and more complicated skills. Her confidence, patience, and upbeat insistence that she's capable of relearning has had positive results beyond what her doctors originally thought possible. Her willingness to accept the limitations that seem to be part of her new normal keeps her from feeling depressed or deprived.

Lasha spoke often about how hearing the voice of her deceased daughter, and also remembering her, gives her the determination and strength to keep fighting, to continue getting better, and to follow her heart in her work and rebuilding her life. Over the years I've spoken with several persons about someone they've loved who has passed on. They've talked of dreaming about the person, having a conversation with their loved one, hearing the person's voice, sensing his or her presence. Many have talked about the influence such encounters have had on their career choices and other decisions made in their lives. We so often hear of encouragement the living give to someone who is faced with an illness, injury, or in treatment. There is no reason to discount the possibility that memories of a departed loved one might offer support and healing to the living. Healing words are as powerful as medicine and offer inspiration for both the body and the soul.

Most of us encounter loss, illness, and unexpected situations, whether with family, with friends, or in our lives. We all need encouragement and words that give us hope and the will to carry on. Lasha shares determination and acceptance of what is lost and also what can be relearned or modified. That determination is the reason Lasha's story is every bit as encouraging and helpful as guidance from a psychiatrist, counselor, wise grandparent, or a religious leader. Encouragement and hope we receive from caring friends, the love of a faithful pet, or the coming of springtime all can contribute to a person's attitude and acceptance, whatever his or her life challenges have been.

1. Lasha's persistence in relearning many actions and information she once knew is admirable and inspiring. How might her story influence your interaction with patients, friends, or family members who have been brain injured, are recovering from a stroke, or are in any situation that has negatively affected their memory?

2. Have you ever experienced temporary or permanent brain damage or worked with people hoping to regain actual brain functions they've lost for various reasons? What stories can you share to inspire others?

3. Many people speak of connecting in some way with loved ones who have died. Some talk of signs they receive. Others sense the presence of a loved one. How do you feel about this aspect of Lasha's story? What can you learn from the experiences others share with you of connecting with a deceased person?

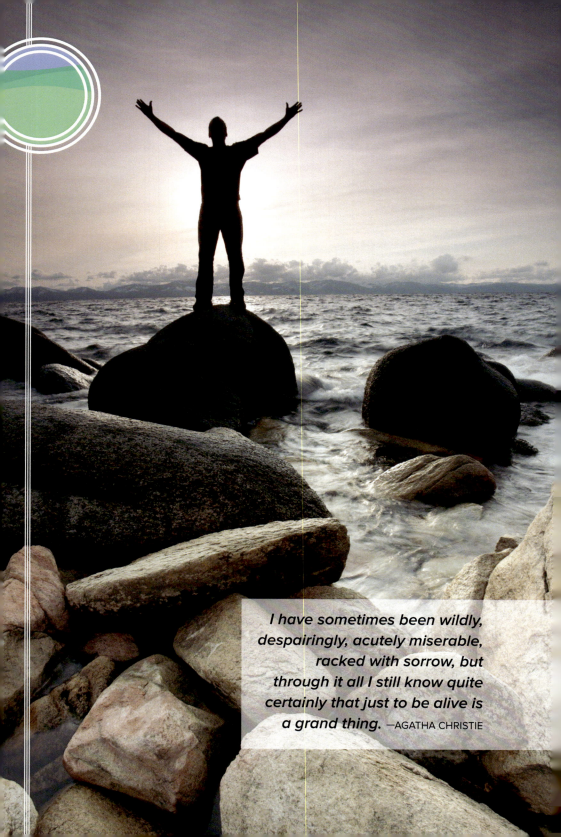

I have sometimes been wildly, despairingly, acutely miserable, racked with sorrow, but through it all I still know quite certainly that just to be alive is a grand thing. —AGATHA CHRISTIE

JEFF
LIVING EACH DAY FULLY

JEFF AND I WERE INTRODUCED VIA E-MAIL THROUGH A FRIEND. She told him I was a collector of stories and asked if he'd be willing to tell me his. "Sure," he said. "Ask her to write to me, and I'll tell her whatever she wants to know."

Jeff had been diagnosed with amyotrophic lateral sclerosis, most often referred to as Lou Gehrig's disease or ALS. He lived with his wife and two young children. Jeff was living locked inside a body that no longer worked. He wouldn't have chosen to be silent, yet he could no longer talk or swallow food, and he had lost an incredible amount of mobility. Jeff had just celebrated his fortieth birthday. He had a birthday cake, but he most likely wasn't able to eat any of it.

Because Jeff and his family live more than two thousand miles from me and he couldn't speak, we never had a phone conversation. Our entire relationship existed through e-mail exchanges. Our friendship grew through honesty and trust. When our correspondence began, Jeff explained in detail how his computer connected him to the world. I learned Jeff was facing new challenges and depreciation almost daily. Yet it was obvious that although Jeff's body could no longer serve him, nothing was wrong with his active, retentive brain. I've combined portions of various e-mail exchanges to give you a presentation with continuity. Here is Jeff's inspiring, life-affirming story in his own words, told between one January and his death in October of the same year.

I'll start my story by telling you about my "can't live without" piece of equipment that has become my mode of communication. My computer allows me to control all functions through my eye movements. I open my e-mail program with my eyes, read the e-mail, then respond by typing with my eyes. There's an on-screen keyboard, and I focus my eyes on a letter or word, and my computer has word prediction capabilities. After I've focused on it for a second, it inserts the letter or word onto the screen. I type with my eyes, and a computerized voice speaks for me. The machine is truly amazing, and it allows me to stay in touch with family and friends and keeps me connected with the world. I can also read the news, do research, and watch my beloved Cincinnati Reds.

Technology is even more amazing than I ever realized. It has enabled me to write things to my children to read after I'm gone. Hopefully, I can teach them some life lessons and give them insights into the person I was. This is important to me, because they're very young now and won't remember much of me. I have so many things I want to tell them.

These days I spend approximately twelve hours a day in my power wheelchair and the other twelve hours in a lift recliner. The power wheelchair allows me to get around, enjoy the warm weather, and attend my children's events. There will come a time when I won't be able to do that, but for now I'm still involved with my kids' activities. My hospital bed isn't comfortable, so I sleep in my lift recliner. So that's some information about my stuff, but here's my story.

I used to be into fitness, going to the gym four to five times a week. I first noticed twitching in my left shoulder, and when it started, I figured it was due to an insufficient amount of potassium. To counteract it, I started eating a lot of bananas. About a month later, I began losing strength very rapidly in my left hand and upper side, my arm, chest, and back. I went to see my general practitioner, and he referred me to a neurologist. He told me that I had two of the three major signs of ALS and referred me to another neurologist for additional testing. My wife and I were constantly researching all the possibilities. We were aware that ALS was a potential diagnosis, but we clung to hope that it was some other disease. With ALS, more often called Lou Gehrig's disease, there is no cure.

Our hope bubble was popped with what felt like an elephant's foot crashing down full force when the doctor told us, "Yes, it's ALS." The memory of first hearing those words remain to still haunt me. My wife and I broke down crying before he finished his last sentence. My thoughts went instantly to the undeniable end result, my death.

Telling my mother and father was one of the most difficult and disheartening things I've ever had to do. I will be their second son to die young. My parents and my other brother will suffer the tragedy of losing another family member. I'll be abandoning my wife and leaving her to raise three small children on her own. Between my bouts of painful sadness, this has all seemed surreal, yet I wasn't in denial. I'd be leaving my children without a father to raise them, celebrate their victories, and console them when they needed it. I was helpless to change the reality, so I began to learn what I needed to live with it.

When I was very early in my deterioration process but still fully functioning, my balance and reaction time were the two things that were affected. One time my kids were in the living room with me, and they started a pillow fight among themselves. I wanted to have fun with them, so I joined in the fracas. My reaction time had become slow and I fell, hitting my head and putting a hole in the wall. I could have fallen on top of one of the kids and injured them. That incident convinced me to also stop driving, not only for my safety, but for the safety of other people too.

The first emotional stage I went through was defiance. I wasn't in denial about having a terminal illness, yet I was determined to fight it. Of course, this was coupled with a good deal of frustration over the loss of functionality that I was experiencing. I distinctly remember combing my daughter's hair and realizing that I no longer had the finger dexterity to give her a ponytail. I definitely wallowed in grief for quite a while after that.

Before long I got to the point where we had to have an elevator installed. This saved us from having to remodel the house, since the full baths are upstairs. I now have a power wheelchair. I can no longer swallow solid food, so I have a feeding tube. Also I've had to step away from more of the things I loved doing—coaching my children's softball team, serving on the board for the local Little League, and being a member of the local school board. Those are the losses that have stung the most.

I now use a cane, foot drop prosthesis, hand splints, extension grabber, elongated shoehorn, zipper pull, buttonhook, and walker. I have several other pieces of equipment. Some I use now, and others I will most likely need soon—a BiPAP machine to help my breathing, cough assist suction for excess saliva, and a Hoyer lift that I'll be forced to use in the future, once my legs can no longer bear my weight. There are also several smaller, less sophisticated pieces, like a shower chair, commode, bidet, a turning wheel for transfers from location to location, and a portable wheelchair.

I felt despair about losing the person I used to be. ALS doesn't care who you once were or how much you fight. It's a nondiscriminating disease that dictates to the person, not the other way around. One thing I've constantly dealt with is frustration about how some people treat me. I've now lost the ability to speak, and many times people see me in a wheelchair and not able to talk, and they treat me as a child. Such situations often give me feelings of hopelessness. I also have constant feelings of loneliness. Even with all the technology that enables me to communicate with my friends and family, they are not real time devices. I am gradually becoming resigned to the fact that, no matter what I do, I will eventually need more help and assistance.

Part of ALS is a side effect called emotional lability. I have a difficult time controlling laughing and or crying. Antidepressants help control this. I spend time each day in meditation, and that calms me down. The most powerful thing that keeps me out of depression is my sweet children. I need to have something to live for beyond myself, and my children are that reason.

Our marriage is a complex relationship that has taken on many different qualities since my symptoms began to appear. Over time it has evolved into a more patient-caregiver relationship. My wife has our three young children to take care of, and takes care of me and also our household. There are only so many hours in the day and the "practical" things need to get taken care of first. This leaves little or no time for us to be husband and wife, nor hardly any time for her to be herself. That being said, she's the person I trust the most with my care. She tells me the way something really is, rather than sugarcoating things.

I have multiple tiers of people who provide my assistance. In tier 1 are the people who provide 24/7 care services to me. Basically, this burden falls almost entirely on my wife. She's the person I call for in the middle of the night, when I need something during the day, or when I want something done that I can't do myself. She's the primary person who handles my feedings and my numerous medications.

I've started pulling my children into support too. They know that Daddy has a muscle problem and that I can't do things for myself. I try to give them age-appropriate tasks, so they're involved. My four-year-old will carry the feeding bag from the kitchen and turn the television off or on for me, and my six-year-old will do those things and also read me her homework, so I can stay involved in that part of their lives. My nine-year-old is getting more involved by moving my hands when necessary, resetting my eye gaze, and moving pieces on my behalf when we play board games.

And then there's tier 2. It includes my home health aide, my parents, my wife's father and his wife of a second marriage, and my brother-in-law. My parents, who don't live near us, have been renting a place locally so they can be close and help out. My wife's family has done the same. Her brother and his wife moved two miles from us, and her father and his wife moved from Florida to be close. The local ALS chapter provides my home health aide. She currently comes here four mornings a week and helps me get ready for the day. This includes brushing and flossing my teeth, shaving my head once a week, shaving my face, showering me, and getting me dressed. In addition to the basic human needs, she also helps by stretching my legs, arms, and neck, and helping make sure I'm set for the day with my computer, TV, or radio. We've been together for a year now, and I trust her implicitly. She knows all my children, my parents, my wife's father and his wife, and some of my friends. Everyone agrees that we hit the lottery when she was assigned to me.

I also have a small handful of friends that I consider tier 3. I confide in them about what is truly happening with me, the extent of the difficulties I face on a daily basis, my mental state, and my worries, hopes, and dreams. These are the few people who truly understand my situation. They serve as my sounding boards and outlets when I want to complain. When they ask how I'm doing, I tell them the truth. I don't put on my public face and say everything is going fine. They don't judge anything I say and also don't tell me what I may want to hear if it's not the truth. I tell them honestly how long I think I have left. We talk about my real fears, not of dying but my fear of my children growing up without a father. We discuss what I can do to help my children understand who I was and what was important to me. Whatever is on my mind or theirs is fair game.

Interestingly, my relationship with each one of these people has grown as a result of the situation. Clearly this is a by-product of spending a lot more time together, yet in some cases it is a result of seeing how willing they are to help. My father is the prime example of someone now doing things that I never thought he would do or could do because he's seventy-four. I've gained a whole new respect for him. I've never felt closer to him than I do now.

Jeff and I carried on a fairly regular e-mail correspondence for a number of months. Then the time between my writing to Jeff and his answers stretched into longer and longer periods. In one of our last e-mail exchanges, I asked him if he'd discuss some of his learning and personal insights that had come to him from dealing with his illness. I share his wise words.

    Knowing there is no hope of recovery has led me to an unexpected freedom. It has enabled me to let go of certain things. I no longer worry about slights or injustices that occurred in the past. I either reconcile them in my mind or just banish them from my thoughts. I don't want to waste any mental energy on negative things. In addition, I now have increased freedom to do what I can and to be whom I choose to be. What I mean is there's no need to play a certain role, as I did when I was healthy, and I feel no pressure to stay in touch with people I'd rather not interact with. At one time I would have done it to be kind and not burn any bridges. Living up to the expectations of others is exhausting. I've been liberated from the conventional wisdom of how a man my age is supposed to behave.

    If a cure for ALS was discovered, would I take it? Certainly I would, yet not to avoid death, but rather to have more of the experience of living. I'm trying to enjoy whatever life I have left. When I think about death, I don't think so much about my physical being. What makes me sad are the things I will miss out on in life. I don't fear death; it's a normal part of the cycle of life. In my situation, there's nothing that I, or anyone, can do about it. My death will come sooner than for some. I was raised Roman Catholic, but I had been questioning religion for quite some time. ALS just speeded up the process. I've now ended up viewing all religions as life philosophies. I take parts from different religions that resonate with me, and I've formed my own guideposts for my beliefs.

    We all have a limited time here on earth, and each of us needs to find the joy in every situation. We all should tell the people we really care about that we love them. While you don't need to make peace with everyone, I'd tell people to let go of old grudges and not waste energy on that stuff. Also, everyone has regrets, but I'd like to tell others they shouldn't spend time or energy focusing on them. You can't change the past, so let it go. I'd let people know they should do things they've always wanted to do, before it gets to be too late or physically impossible.

Some people don't deal well with illness. Don't hold that against them. I, and others, have a chance to educate people, especially children, about how to deal with people with disabilities. Embrace the opportunity, let them ask questions and touch equipment, and deal with situations realistically. This will be part of a lasting legacy you can leave behind for others. If you can write or speak or somehow document your life, leave your life lessons for others. It will be a way for others to know who you were and what in your life mattered most to you. And most important, tell people you love them and how much they mean to you.

I now understand why some people have an urge to give things away as they get older. Whether its money or material possessions, I've found that they truly don't matter in the scheme of things. So if I can create a memory, make someone happy, or leave a remembrance by giving someone something of mine, then that is the best use of one of my physical items that I can think of.

Since losing my voice, I have a newfound appreciation for listening more to others. I have learned so much more by listening than I ever did by talking. If I had it to do all over again, I would focus more on the quality of experiences over quantity in everything. So there you have it, except for one more thing I want to say.

I have some of the most amazing people in my life: my wife, my children, other family and friends. Someone is always around to brighten my day with a smile, give me a laugh, or help me with whatever I may need. My dad has been there for me every day. He has been my chauffeur, nurse, waiter, personal shopper, handyman, debate colleague, news source, and a ton of other things, depending on what I need. He has been my number one champion and friend. Thanks, Dad, for everything. I love you.

In the final week of our correspondence, I wrote Jeff three short e-mails, sent a "thinking of you" card to his home, and began editing my collection of Jeff's e-mails, so I could share with others the strength of character and the insights he had discovered. What turned out to be the last e-mail from Jeff arrived.

My apologies for not responding earlier. I don't do a lot of e-mail anymore. As expected, my body has continued to decline, and I'm finding that dying a prolonged death is tiring. Keeping up the fight is getting wearisome. I have a bookmark that has a quote on it from Nathaniel Hawthorne. If I remember correctly, it reads, "May you live every day of your life." Since coming to terms with my impending death, I use this saying almost as a personal motto. I would tell others to be present in whatever situation they're in. Rather than focusing on death, I still try to focus on living. Maybe my thoughts could help others in some way deal with whatever they're facing or dealing with in their lives.

Less than a month later someone in Jeff's family sent me his obituary. Jeff's adjusting to and accepting his life-changing medical diagnosis and the expectancy of a drastically shortened life brought with it major life changes and a totally changed perspective. His busy, goal-oriented world quickly faded when ALS became the primary focus of his life.

I saw in his e-mails that through his illness the importance of material things and related goals quickly diminished. He learned the true value of living each day. Hopefully, Jeff's story can teach all of us, whether we're the caregiver or the one receiving care, that both our bodies and our thinking change as time passes. We don't necessarily need illness to motivate us to reflect on what is meaningful and lasting in our lives. I often quote an observation I heard the Minnesota senator and former Vice President Hubert Humphrey offer in an interview after his cancer surgery: "Oh, my friend, it's not what they take away from you that counts. It's what you do with what you have left."

1. Relatively healthy people can unexpectedly find they have a fatal disease or some life-changing prognosis. A happy, busy life can also be turned around suddenly by an accident or diagnosis. How could you help, comfort, and offer perspective to someone dealing with such an unexpected situation?

2. Have any of your family members, friends, or clients needed help with physical decline? How have you handled this? How have they responded? How might you offer help in a way that is less likely to elicit a response such as "I can do it myself"?

3. Have you had a life-changing event or diagnosis in your own life? If so, what have you learned, either as the one in care or the caregiver, that can you offer to others?

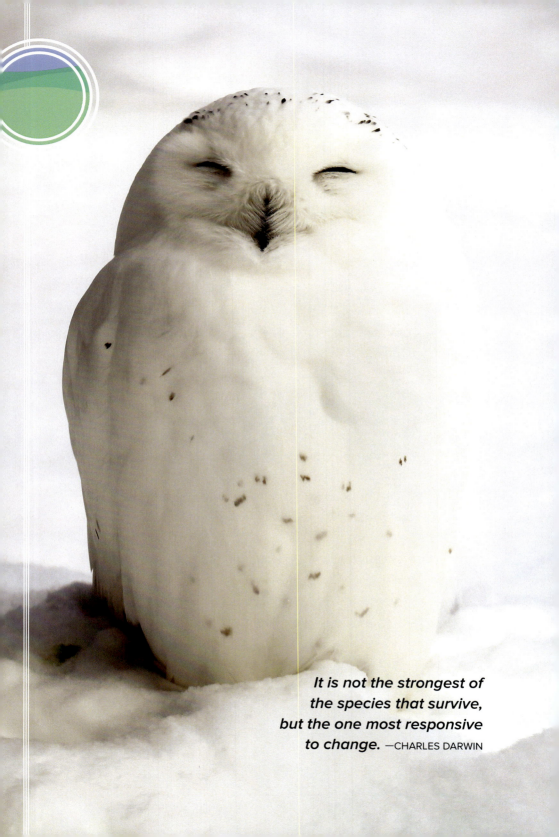

It is not the strongest of the species that survive, but the one most responsive to change. —CHARLES DARWIN

SUZ
LIFE IN A SUPPORT COMMUNITY

YES, HER NAME IS SUSAN, BUT SHE PREFERS TO BE CALLED SUZ. She now is sixty-five years old and living with a diagnosis of stage 4 cancer. She describes her life as a wild ride. She was a political activist for many years, was married, and went back to school because she had a lust for learning. She trained as a clinical psychologist and worked at a psychiatric unit at the university. Eventually Suz came to a point where she didn't feel satisfied with that work and wanted to be outdoors. She also came to realize that she really loved being with children and enjoyed animals too. That changed her direction totally. Suz went to work for a program on a farm that teaches children who need psychological and behavioral help to care for others with compassion and understanding. She also began doing that training with many groups all over the world.

Very close to where I live there's a private cancer center that doesn't offer cures but provides abundant comfort. Two people who had cancer founded this center about twenty years ago. The atmosphere is warm and full of positive energy. The center offers a variety of supportive activities along with sincere caring and love. All the activities and groups are available to area residents and also their families and close friends. There's real love there. Facing my days has become part of who I am and how I live with my eventual dying.

My husband and I are divorced, and I live alone with my dog. My little private house is at the edge of the woods, and I'm surrounded by abundant natural growth. I have dealt with multiple myeloma for seven years. It's really one of the worst cancers a person can have. It eats away at my bone marrow, and my bones are extremely fragile now. If I were to bend over to paint my toenails or pick something up, I'd probably crack a rib. My cancer is just part of who I am now, though. What I mean is that I don't wake up every morning and think something like, "Oh, my God, I've got cancer!" That would get me into some dark spiral. Instead, I think things like, "My dog wants to go out, so I'll get up now," or I plan what am I'm going to do today.

I belong to a group of people at the center who meet to work toward accepting our new normal and living each day in a conscious way. We all have been diagnosed with different cancers, but each has been told we were in stage 4. We call our group Living Well with Incurable Cancer. The center, what I call a haven and a blessing, is in a beautiful building and offers all kinds of healing services to people who have cancer. There are scheduled yoga, exercise, and small meeting groups; free counseling; singing; instruction on cooking healthy food; meditation; and many other services. The focus of everything is on living.

A lot of support is offered to teach us how to be with our cancer, and a contagious healing power is alive when we're in our group. It's not about healing the cancer, but we're learning how to let our fears and our feelings come up and come out.

We each make an effort to turn away from fear and into the energy to live each day. You could say in one sentence that I, and my small group, support a healing that allows us to just be with the reality of our illness. We're trying not to fix it but to accept it and live consciously each day. That's not a bad idea for anyone, whether the person has an illness or is active and well, right? I try to live fully and value and appreciate each day. It's a philosophy that keeps me in the present.

I remember waking up in the hospital seven years ago and telling my oncologist that I was going to fight my cancer my way. People have many different sources of strength and inspiration for their spiritual path. Some call it God, Spirit, Higher Power, or whatever evokes a deep connection within themselves. I have a spiritual practice of meditation that has been part of my life for many years now.

These days when I'm really in pain, crying, and feeling physically weak, I lift my head up and pray or think of my deeper connection to a Higher Power. Then slowly, somehow the pain begins to subside and fade away. Precancer, I would want to speak to someone or try to include another person in my experience. Now my spiritual practice grows inside me and is private. How shall I say it? Perhaps with the blessing of cancer I've become deeply in touch with these feelings inside myself that have both spiritual and religious connections. I say "blessing" because the cancer experience has actually been a gift that has made my spiritual connection more personal and deeply meaningful. It's like turning my small self over to my Higher Power. That's the best way I can explain it. So the path of my cancer is out of my hands.

Others have an attachment to some established religious faith. I also know people whose religion is the beauty of becoming completely immersed in nature and the outdoors.

It's what feeds their inner self. For others, their support comes from deep connections to family and their friends. That human connection is their inspiration and their strength to deal with their illness in a life-affirming way. The best way I can describe it is that we all choose our own way, and those in my group are respectful of that.

I've made a related observation about the changes that come to a body that is aging, let alone one with a disease like cancer. I don't think our culture easily accepts the natural aging process. It seems to me that living long term with a cancer diagnosis has similarities to living with an aging body, even for a person who is relatively healthy. Our spirits can stay healthy, vibrant, and full, even if our bodies can't keep up the old ways, whether we have an illness or are just experiencing aging. Clutching and holding on to the person we once were doesn't really work. The body has its own process, and it changes as the years pass. So, some days aren't good for me, but I know I can help my outlook change. We all can learn how to do that.

What I'm saying is that I work at living in the present. When my body is feeling pain, I don't go to the future or the past by saying, "What's wrong? I was doing so well yesterday." I stay with what is happening in the present. For me, that's very healing. I see that in my group we help each other acknowledge that all of life is really one day at a time, and we have to live in that day. I don't think we understand "one day at a time" deeply until the day something comes into our life and forces us to learn that, and to come to understand that we really can, and must, live that way. Today is all each of us has now. I didn't know that before. I used to be always striving to get more, do better, get ahead somehow, and now I really understand I wasn't really living life in its fullness. I've only grown into this new awareness as I've learned to live with my cancer.

I'm with people who also have found a way to live in their cancer. We each need to seek out people who are on a similar path of learning and who are growing into a new way of living for themselves as changes come into our lives. It's critical to have that support, and we need people in our lives who get it. That's the best way I can find to say it. If you can find such connections, your journey will be a good deal easier. Some might see me living a limited life, yet my view is that each of my days is deep and meaningful.

> *I will do something today that will make me feel that I have really lived this day.* —ANONYMOUS

Suz describes her deeply meaningful connection with self, and others, through her practice of meditation. Many people have expressed in their own way a deepening of such feelings within themselves and those around them. She talks of a deeper attachment to a supreme power and to the people who share her life. Many I've talked with at various times have shared a personal relationship with a power that gives them both strength and comfort. For many, including Suz, and possibly each of us in our own way, such a connection is a source of strength as we travel our paths.

Suz has no wish for miracles. Her hope is to live in a meaningful way, knowing that her cancer cannot be cured and that her days are limited. Yet in our conversation she made sure I understood that her intentions and her actions focus on living. She offers me and others an understanding of acceptance, spiritual strength, and the blessings we all have by realizing we all can live only one day at a time.

My conversation with Suz brought to mind my visit with a woman who could move only with her wheelchair. She told me that before I arrived to talk with her, she had sat in her small garden for over four hours and watched a flower open. I will always remember what she said about that experience. "As the flower opened, an awareness rose deep inside me. It was as deep, comforting, accepting, and beautiful as the flower." Both the woman who watched the flower open and Suz understand that we have an inner self to discover.

Our conversation got me thinking about a quote from Mitch Albom's book *Tuesdays with Morrie:* "I give myself a good cry if I need it. But then I concentrate on the good things still in my life. I don't allow myself any more self-pity than that. A little each every morning, a few tears, and that's all." Then he talks about filling the rest of his day with living his life. Suz offers a similar message. I don't throw the word *wisdom* around randomly; yet, in my opinion, this philosophy that both Morrie and Suz embraced is deep wisdom.

1. **As changes have come into your life, have you found a new community or helped create a group that offers mutual understanding and support? Recall a story that you experienced or that others have shared with you.**

2. **What support and guidance do you receive from a particular religion or spiritual practice, such as meditation, deep reflection, or silent retreats? What challenges or struggles have you faced personally or with family members or clients? How have they helped you grow in your philosophies and beliefs?**

3. **What inner rewards have you or someone you know discovered in slowing the pace of your life? Recall a story that tells of growth and understanding of a new depth of personal acceptance. How have you held on to those insights?**

SANDRA
FINDING OPTIMISM AND PEACE

You have to count on living every single day in a way you believe will make you feel good about your life, so if it were over tomorrow, you'd be content. —JANE SEYMOUR

MOST PEOPLE WHO MOVE INTO A RETIREMENT COMMUNITY aren't as young as Sandra and her husband, Bill, were when they made that decision. Over 90 percent of persons in their sixties want to live in their own homes as long as possible. Yet when Sandra and Bill faced a dramatic change in her health, they decided the move was the perfect choice for them. She was sixty-two, and Bill was sixty-one. For over a dozen years they've now called a comfortable and friendly retirement residence their home.

When Sandra learned I was collecting stories that could be inspiring to others, she wanted to tell me her personal story. Many people offer to share their experiences because they feel they may be a source of comfort to someone else. Her religion is one of the strengths she relies upon, but she knows that her attitude toward her physical problems makes a great difference too. I enjoyed meeting Sandra and sharing a conversation and a cup of tea. As she requested, I'm sharing some of the inspiration of her story with you.

We made the decision to move into this retirement residence when it was evident I would no longer be able to manage in our two-story home. We were both in our early sixties, somewhat younger than most who live here. We're in our seventies now. This location is not too far from where my daughter is living. Our two sons and their families live much farther away, but I'm in touch with them pretty often. When we moved here my husband hadn't retired yet, so he went to work every day. Now he's left the work world and he rides his bike, snowshoes in the winter, hikes, and walks our dog. He's got high blood pressure and diabetes, but he's active and busy, and he takes good care of himself and of me.

Living in this retirement community is fine for me. My husband and I both appreciate the atmosphere and the services that are available. We don't want to shovel snow any longer or mow the lawn and all that. Many personal services are available right here, like getting my haircut and a manicure, and the meals are good too. Some people don't like the idea of living in a retirement residence, but we enjoy the many benefits.

Nine years ago I was diagnosed with kidney cancer and was lucky enough to qualify to get a kidney transplant. After the surgery, although no medical person has been able to describe to me exactly what happened, my vision was badly affected.

I'm now legally blind. I've been in a wheelchair for over twelve years. I used a walker at first, but when my eyesight failed completely, I did better in a wheelchair. The doctors think the kidney transplant may have brought the loss of my sight, but it's never been confirmed. However, if I hadn't had the kidney transplant, I would have died then. Although it's been a number of years, I've had a reoccurrence of the kidney cancer. It's in my other kidney now. I may face pain in the future, but I have peace inside. Thankfully, I've come to this time in my life with a readiness to deal with it.

Seven years after we were married our lives were a mess. My husband and I used to have a group of friends that drank a lot and very often. It used to be our way of enjoying ourselves and handling things. That behavior had become excessive, and we realized it. I don't want to talk about specifics, but our lives became complicated.

I was unhappy and confused, and I started to go to church. That was thirty years ago, much earlier in our lives. The children were young, we joined the church, the kids went to Bible classes, and our religious beliefs became the center of family life. As we didn't drink anymore, we no longer spent time with our old friends. Our lives changed and new people and activities came into our lives. Religion isn't the answer for everyone, but it became a comfort and a support that I'd never had before. I now have a peace that goes beyond whatever happens in my life.

I've seen that people who don't have anything to hold on to are terribly bitter, somehow desperate and depressed. I don't mean they lack possessions and physical things. They haven't come to a place where they can live with however things are for them at this moment. You know, people can get so tied up in their own things, so focused on themselves, that they're unaware of others. Some people get angry and never get out of it, and don't see anything good in their lives or out in the world. I don't know how others come to a place of acceptance, but for me, it's my religion. It's within me, deeply within me. Religion isn't everyone's belief and strength. There are many paths to peace of mind and acceptance of the challenges in life. But for me, religion has changed everything.

When I get together with a group of women here at the home, they often talk about their problems. Each of them is hurting and sometimes frightened of what they have to deal with. I try to encourage them to find a comfortable way to live with their challenge. I tell them that my personal solution is my religion and my beliefs. I know others need to look elsewhere for their personal way of facing their health challenges and unexpected changes in their lives. People need to find their own path to acceptance of their reality and an appreciation and awareness of every day of their life.

Now I'm facing a new cancer in my kidney and I'm in a wheelchair. The people around me can see how relaxed and accepting I am, and I sincerely believe I'll be able to face whatever is ahead in my life. People tell me that I smile a lot, and I guess I am truly happy. Maybe the word that best describes me is *peaceful*. As I think about it now, the word I'd choose to explain myself is *content*. Yes, I'm content, and I truly understand the joy of living one day at a time.

> *It takes courage to grow up and turn out to be who you really are.* —E. E. CUMMINGS

I will remember Sandra as a woman who wouldn't let disability define her. I've encountered others who did the opposite. I'm sure many of us have too. Many people allow the loss of a limb, the limitation of an aging body, or the diagnosis of a disease that changes the planned course of their lives to leave them feeing helpless and hopeless. Some fight it like an enemy they can conquer; others live with the changes and modify their path.

As different as each human is from another, so the way we adjust to changes in our lives, both small and large, is individual. We learn to deal with changes or challenges we choose, and also those that are unplanned or unexpected. I often wonder about the life rafts we choose when our normal responses no longer fit the situation. I've reflected how differently I've reacted at different times in my life to various situations and challenges that unexpectedly come into my life or that of a loved one. Both the attitude and the actions taken as we deal with our particular situations influence the outcome.

Sandra's story is an invitation to look at my own story, to truly assess what gives me peace, optimism, and the emotional strength needed to make tough decisions and hold the confidence that has grown within me. I hope it might put others on that path too. We each make personal choices that we hope will help us find a way to nurture our inner strengths. Many choose a religious path as Sandra has. Others have built their attitudes, behaviors, and values on different philosophies or beliefs. The gift of Sandra's story leaves us with the challenge to focus on our own strengths and beliefs, to nurture ourselves, and to accept our health and behavior changes so we continue to grow in depth, compassion, and wisdom.

1. Letting go of a family home and a familiar neighborhood and moving into a retirement community is a personal and often difficult decision. When have you seen such a decision result in a positive outcome for both the people who made the move and their family too?

2. What can you do to help yourself and others realize and accept that life is about change? How can a realistic acceptance of a life change help your families and others adjust to those challenges?

MARCUS
A NEW NORMAL

I want to go home and make a difference in the world. —SUSIE SMITH

THOSE RETURNING FROM SERVICE IN THE ARMED FORCES FACE a multitude of adjustments to civilian life. Every story that veterans either tell or keep hidden remains part of their past and their future. Thousands of combat experiences—many tragic, some brave and hopeful—have been shared, although others may never be revealed. Yet like all the other stories in this book, this one may offer the reader a new insight or awareness and also inspire empathy and support.

This story is about Marcus, a now thirty-seven-year-old veteran of the Iraq War. I had a conversation with him in his warm and welcoming home built for him by Homes for Our Troops, a nonprofit organization that empowers wounded war vets and their families.

Marcus and the woman who became his wife two years ago enjoy a quiet, rural view from their comfortable, accessible home. He and his dog welcomed me at their front door; physically handicapped, Marcus walked more slowly than the pup. When we were seated at his dining room table, he started to share his story.

I had been working in retail management for about five years, and I wanted to do something that had more purpose, to help others in some way. I thought I'd apply to be a firefighter, but I didn't have any training that would fit the requirements, someone with either military training or medical education. I thought about that and decided if I joined the military and trained as a medic, I could get an education in both of those fields. I wasn't a believer in the war, but many young people were going overseas, putting their lives at risk in Iraq. They often were getting wounded, and I believed I would be able to help them.

I went through basic training and also got advanced medical training as a combat medic. I was told that I would be assigned to a unit in Iraq. Shortly after I got there, a roadside bomb hit the truck I was in. The truck went into the air maybe twenty-five to thirty feet and landed upside down. I was next to the driver, and he was killed. I was unconscious, and when I woke up five days later, I was in a hospital in Germany. I had a broken jaw, and I couldn't open my mouth or talk. I also had two broken legs, and both feet were broken too. I had a burst spleen, a fractured left arm, a brain injury, and post-traumatic stress disorder. I had a lot of healing ahead, and no one made me any promises. I had many, many surgeries. I don't even remember how many. I was in and out of a wheelchair. That was more than ten years ago.

I was lucky to have a lot of support, and I trusted my doctors. I did everything they told me to do. I trusted they knew more about my injuries than I did. I guess I was able to not be angry like some vets might have been. Most of the time, I was able to make the best of my situation. A psychiatrist told me that I had an ability to compartmentalize, to not continually focus on my disabilities and losses but to appreciate that I was alive and healing. Sure, I had, and still have, some down days. Some of those times were really tough. But I didn't have a seriously lasting depression. I think that helped me to participate actively in my recovery.

I want to say something about having family that's supportive and tell you about the unexpected help I had through it all. I was transferred to a hospital in the United States, and my younger brother was able to come and live near me and help me full time. One year before my injury he had fallen off a roof and has been left with serious injuries. He was healed enough to look for a job, and the army created a job for him as a caregiver for me. They offered to pay my brother eighty-five dollars a day to be at the hospital and serve as full-time help for me. He could take me to medical appointments, do practical and helpful things like push my wheelchair around, and be my moral support. Having him with me kept my attitude positive. Having someone in my family there with me gave me a very personal and meaningful kind of support. Of course, having around-the-clock help was important, but that my brother was the one doing those things for me was a special comfort to me and for the rest of my family too.

I remember after one of my many surgeries when I was taken back to my room. I was in a great deal of pain, and my attitude was bad. My brother came into my room smiling and upbeat, and I was angry and depressed and very verbal about it. He got a serious look on his face and said some magic words. "You know, whenever you have pain or something traumatic in your life, you have a choice. Either you can get bitter, or you can get better." That helped me to check myself and know that I had a choice.

As for my situation now, I never know if and when I'll need more surgeries. I'm pretty sure that at some point along the way, one of my feet will need to be amputated. My arthritis is getting much worse, and I'm getting new and strange feelings in my legs, and my back has started to have all kinds of pains and discomfort. When I got out of bed this morning I felt my right arm was okay, but my left arm was heavy. I suspect something is wrong there. I don't know what's ahead, but they're doing great things with prosthetics these days, and that's in my favor.

When I was in Iraq, I was looking ahead to coming back home and thinking about some kind of work or study program that would give me training to become a nurse. After both of my feet were so badly injured, that was no longer in the cards for me. I asked myself what my goals were for when I recovered. I kept thinking something like, get a place to call home, buy a truck, get a dog, and go back to school. I also kept thinking a lot about a soldier I knew who committed suicide. At his funeral I was aware how terribly sad the circumstances of his death were and thought that maybe it could have been prevented. It made me aware that maybe I could do something to help prevent this happening to others. If I dedicated my life to this, it would be a worthy cause. It could help many veterans and their families. I did some research and found that social work would be an appropriate area of study.

When I was back home and healed enough, I went back to college to study sociology. I'm happy to tell you that I've already got my bachelor's degree, and I'm just about to get my graduate degree. My thesis is a research project on the effects of mindfulness practice on post-traumatic stress disorder and brain injury. I hope to work mostly with vets. There's really a need there, and I want those problems to be attended to. I'm one veteran who's willing and able to take on that challenge.

I often think about how I was very lucky to get help both in my family and with professionals who listened to me and helped me deal with my feelings. Even though I'm aware that I'll continue to need help and support, I'm ready to offer my support to others. I can help vets find ways to talk it out and not keep those painful memories and fears inside. You can't change the truth of something that has happened to you, but each person needs to find a way to work it through and not keep it in a place that prevents healing and a decent life. Many vets need a comrade, a friend, family members, or a professional—someone trusted who can really understand and empathize. Sometimes a family member can't deal with those stories, but I can. That's the way I want to live and be available to others. A vet living with emotions, memories, or an uncertain future and then choosing suicide is tragic.

I'm confident that I can maintain a positive attitude, and I can help others adopt a life-affirming view of their lives. I've got a job to do. I trust I'll continue to get what care I need. I had a positive attitude before I got hurt, and that has contributed to my resilience. I was fortunate to have friends and family and professional help who were supportive and stayed by me. Many in service have had negative and distressing experiences. They live with memories and fears that can make all the difference in a person's quality of life. It also can have an impact on those they live with. It's also often difficult to help someone change a hopeless, tortured, and negative attitude.

Yet the people in our lives, the people we're in close relationships with and whom we trust, can offer nonjudgmental listening and hopefully contribute to the healing process.

When your life is almost taken, almost totally lost, you look at what's important for each day of your life. I've spent a good deal of time doing that, and I realize for me, what matters is spending time with people I can help, being with those I love, enjoying whatever new experiences I can have—like going hunting and fishing—and finding any excuse to stay in touch with others. I'm enjoying my life and appreciating it. I'll continue to use my attitude, my experience, and my desire to help others. If you asked me how things are going for me, I'd say, "My life is good."

> *Through the experience of trial and suffering, the soul can be strengthened, ambition inspired and success be achieved.* —HELEN KELLER

I was surprised when I heard Marcus say at the conclusion of our conversation that his life is good. Although he's living with the reality of pain, limitations, and uncertainty, he embraces the positives in each day. Marcus looks ahead with a sense of purpose. This appreciation for being alive is, regrettably, not present in the lives of many survivors and their families.

For more than twenty years PTSD (post-traumatic stress disorder) has been understood as a mental disorder. Veterans who have been in war zones are often deeply troubled by what they've seen and experienced, yet many are not seeking or receiving the emotional, mental, and physical support they need. Some are reluctant to talk with family or even close friends about comrades who were wounded or died and other horrors of war they witnessed. Very often veterans hide their apprehensions and fears, both consciously and unconsciously, to protect themselves and to avoid hurting others. Reentering civilian life and adjusting to the ambitions and values of our culture can be an uncomfortable challenge, and for some impossible. Many veterans and others whose lives have been changed drastically from war, disease, or accident have not come to a place of acceptance with their new situation. Regrettably, some veterans choose not to continue living, yet others are able to adjust in some ways and carry on.

Healing and adjusting for both veterans and close family needs to begin with honest, deeply empathetic conversation. A vet may need months, even years, to reveal painful memories. Each individual's experience is, of course, vastly different from another's. Some returning veterans might be open to conversation with a therapist, social worker, minister, rabbi or clergy of another religious affiliation. A struggling vet might be willing to talk with parents, siblings, a spouse, or other close family member or trusted friend.

I can only hope that this story speaks to both family caregivers and those in care. It's vital that the government continues to offer financial support and personal help to veterans. Returning service persons very often need the help, support, and patience of families and communities. We can come to learn from others as they share their stories and encourage veterans and their families to seek necessary help.

1. Have you had an experience in your family with a returning veteran? If so, what is this person willing to talk about, and what situations or feelings does he or she not discuss? What help could you offer?

2. Has anyone in your family or someone you know been diagnosed with PTSD? What symptoms have you observed, such as inappropriate conversation or other behavior suggesting undiagnosed PTSD?

3. What has this story given you to think about—possibly some fear or feeling or even an undiscovered strength?

4. How might you offer support to a returning veteran in your neighborhood or someone you know?

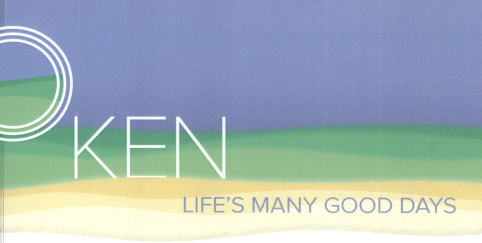

KEN
LIFE'S MANY GOOD DAYS

How do we live so that we shape our legacy consciously, so that the best of who we are and what we value lives on? —MEG NEWHOUSE

MANY PEOPLE SPEND THEIR LAST DAYS IN A HOSPITAL OR facility that provides hospice services. Hospice care is for people approaching death. Hospice services are offered in several locations and in a variety of situations, and can also be provided at home. Always, it emphasizes life. Ken had been in hospice home care for several months when we talked. That arrangement allowed him to continue living in his own familiar and comfortable home. He died in his own bed with his springer spaniel by his side, as was his choice.

Several weeks before his death, Ken and I had a conversation as we sat on his deck overlooking the river he loved. We talked about what his life had been and what it had become. Although he was no longer able to practice law, his work life and reputation had earned him many awards and national visibility. Over decades he had fought for civil and personal rights and also had been a mentor to many law students. He was known and is remembered as a champion of justice for all.

The day we talked was sunny and warm, and we ate lunch outside under the table umbrella. Ken relished the simple things every day of the life he had left. We celebrated that day with ice cream for dessert. I didn't even ask him a question. He just began telling me what he was living with at that moment.

My body has deteriorated a good deal. I have a pacemaker, an artificial heart valve, and a repaired heart valve. I've had congestive heart failure, and that causes urine retention. My COPD, a chronic lung disorder, was diagnosed more than eighteen years ago. Every year at my checkup, the specialist tells me, "It's just a little bit worse." That means I now have both heart and lung disease, which means limited lung capacity and extremely shallow breathing. I also have limited kidney function, poor hearing, and reduced mobility. I'm pretty exhausted after taking very few steps. I no longer get enjoyment out of eating even a beautifully prepared meal, but I do like ice cream, and I eat that every day. I get pleasure from visits from many lawyers, past clients, and neighbors, and my large family. I have five middle-aged children (the oldest is sixty-four), twenty-five grandchildren, and thirty-five great grandchildren.

What really has been hard for me these past few months has been giving up the independence of my regular daily routine. Today my back aches, there's a pain running down my right leg, and I'm very, very fatigued. My breathing is heavy, and I'm coughing a lot. I want to keep doing whatever I can for myself, but on a day like today, I'll take any help that's offered. You know, I can't do normal things like lift something heavy or tie my shoes; doing things like that totally exhausts me. I immediately have to rest for a while or sleep. People are surprised at what I can do, but after I do it, I have to call it quits and maybe sleep an hour.

I need whoever helps me to understand how important it is for me to be involved in the decisions about that help. You need somebody there to help you when you need it, but it's important for my helper to understand that I can think and talk and participate in decisions about my care. The nurses from hospice understand that, and so does a woman who is here four hours a day to help in the house and with whatever I need. She and I play a lot of gin rummy. She's a pretty aggressive card player, and she doesn't let me win just because I'm an old, sick guy. I have to concentrate on the game, because she's tough, and I need that.

The woman I've loved and lived with for several years now is my full-time caregiver. I get pleasure out of having her in my life. She lets me try to do many things by myself. I appreciate that, because I don't like the feeling of being dependent. I was very depressed at first, but now I know how to live this life, and I've adjusted pretty well.

Being in court or working on a legal case took sixteen to eighteen hours a day of energy and involvement, so I gave up my law practice, because that wasn't possible any longer. Eventually I gave up my teaching in the law school, because I no longer felt I had the energy to instill a passion in my students that would change their lives. I no longer had either good hearing or the capacity to speak loudly enough to do the kind of teaching that would deepen a person. It's not just words that teach students; it was also the atmosphere of my classes, the deep learning, and the power I was able to offer my students. My passion has been the law, and I knew how to create that passion in my students. My way of teaching isn't lectures so much as student involvement. But my loss of hearing was so drastic that I couldn't continue that way of running my classes. In every aspect of my life I was responsible and in charge, and now that's impossible. I now lack the energy and the capacity to make the same contributions to society I used to.

All my children and my grandchildren too try to include me and encourage me to come along to various events, but I just can't do those things anymore, even with their help. They always say things like, "Come on, we'll help you. We'll do everything." They're sincere and eager to include me, but I can't walk more than a few steps. They don't want to see that reality.

I look around at others who are out in the world in a way I can no longer handle, and I think they should be working to make our world a safer and more just society. I want to leave something behind to make this world a little bit better. I'm not talking only about a personal legacy of family values, but whatever I can do to make the world a better place for those who aren't as fortunate as I am. These priorities haven't changed since I was a young man, but what I can actually do about those priorities has changed drastically now. I've always felt that I need to live my life in a way that balances my obligations to myself, to my family, to those who need guidance and help, and to the world. My family—my partner, and my children—each in her or his own way, have the same values.

On days when I get angry and frustrated about what's going on with my body, I keep hoping these problems will disappear. If I can ignore these physical disabilities and not focus on them, I find I'm much better off. What I've discovered is that the difference between a good day and a bad day for me is basically what I do with it in my head. I've put a lot of energy into unlearning the "poor me" attitude. However, it was a hard lesson for me to accept my limitations. I'll tell you the story of how I learned what wasn't possible for me anymore.

Every summer for many years a close friend and I would captain a boat in the Caribbean, where we'd sail together to many of the islands. When I was the captain of the boat, I was in charge of everything. When he died I could no longer manage to sail alone, so I gave up trying to captain a boat any longer. It was hard to let that part of my life end. My next trips, for as long as I felt I could get on and off a sailboat easily, I went sailing with someone else taking the captain role.

Last summer I accepted an invitation to go on a sailing trip in the Caribbean Islands with my son and his wife. The woman I now share my life with suspected it would be too difficult for me, but I had always been so happy on a boat, and I was confident I could handle the trip. My son was trained to captain the boat, and we would just be guests, not crew. All we'd have to do was enjoy sitting on the deck, sleep in our bunks at night, and get out of the boat at the different places when we would dock.

I had a wheelchair in the airport, so that was easy, and we flew to our destination. I was okay until we got to the boat dock and had a really long walk to get to our boat. That first challenge gave me an indication that I was in trouble. Walking the length of the dock was exhausting and very, very slow. Then I had a good deal of trouble getting onto the boat. It was humiliating for me in its difficulty, and I remembered how easy it had been for so many years of sailing. Getting around inside the boat was much too hard for me, so I sat in one place, and going to the bathroom during the night was difficult too. When the others went up to sit on the deck, I was too worn out to join them.

My exhaustion showed me that the trip wasn't going to be possible for me. After one night on the boat, I asked my son to take us to a hotel on shore. He and his wife continued on their sailing trip, and we flew home the next morning. It became obvious to me after one night on the boat that I had taken my last sailing trip. I had let my wishes ignore my reality. It was a sad thing for me after my many years of sailing. I had hoped that if I could just make it onto the boat, the biggest challenge would have been handled. I wasn't facing the reality of my limitations. I had loved to sail, but I'm too limited now to do that anymore. That experience was my real learning about both my current limitations and my increasing disability. This experience made me considerably more willing to accept help.

Now, I'm more dependent as the weeks go by. It's so annoying to have to wait until my partner or someone comes around to help. I sit there waiting, wishing I could do whatever it is or get whatever I want for myself. Many small things, little meaningless tasks, exhaust me these days, and it makes me both angry and sad. I don't mind at all asking others to do the big things. It's the smaller things that often exhaust me so much these days, so I'm learning how to ask for help. I'm also noticing that whoever is around and gets me a glass of water or the newspaper often says something like, "I'm glad you asked." I never realized there were satisfactions in both giving and getting help. It goes both ways.

I feel a bit worse every day, and I've come to accept that reality. What I'm saying is that I've now cut my expectations down to the reality. It's like a child whose eyes are bigger than his stomach. I've frequently bit off more than I can chew. I'll say it like this: I have to take little bites of activity, such as walking up the driveway to the mailbox, and then I have to take a significant rest.

It's summer now, and I sit outside most of every day and look at the river. My home overlooks the river, and it's peaceful and gives me great pleasure. Nothing is better than the river I live on. It says to me that it's a beautiful world out there. We humans have an obligation to preserve that beauty and the preciousness of nature's world. I hope people will realize what we all have and how vital it is that we work to preserve it.

I'm not afraid of death. I think more about my growing dependency and how I'm going to handle that. I think what people fear is the process of dying. This may sound rather silly, but I think about my funeral and what people might say. I'd like to hover over that event and hear what they're saying.

I had a dream about dying last night. It didn't frighten me, because at this stage of my life and my deteriorated health, I'm going to either live a little longer before I die or live a little shorter and die. In the dream it was my funeral, and what frightened me was that no one came. Death doesn't scare me, but my dream made me unhappy. I want my family and friends and all those I've worked with and lived with in my lifetime to remember what my life stood for. I don't want the things they remember about me to be particularly personal. I want to think that I've left a legacy of fighting for justice and social equity. My fights have been beyond superficialities. I'm proud of my work and my teaching. I've only one life to give to the cause of empowering individuals and communities, and I hope many others will pick up where I've left off.

> **At the end of my life, I would hope that I would not have a single bit of talent left, and could say, "I used everything you gave me."** —ERMA BOMBECK

My conversation with Ken left me thinking about two important subjects: accepting care and leaving a legacy. A person dealing with terminal illness and the need for help from another has to make unexpected and unwanted compromises. In such situations a person rarely recovers uncompromised independence. Ken's dramatic experience with the sailing trip that he had so much anticipated and already embarked upon was a difficult way to learn to accept his growing number of limitations.

I hope others might avoid such a major incident by accepting their advancing dependence. I know of several people who have fallen and broken a leg or hip, or suffered some other injury because of an "I can do it myself" attitude. A caregiver can ease each necessary letting go by recognizing the independence remaining and offering the support, understanding, and caring that eases the letting go. For a caregiver to offer sympathetic and empathetic understanding and to help the person in care to still feel in charge of his or her own life is a major challenge.

The other important and vital insight I gained from the conversation with Ken was about our yearning to leave a legacy. He didn't talk about his physical possessions, his property, or his will. He talked at some length about what people had learned from the way he lived his life and how it might nurture theirs. When each of us departs this life, we leave to others the memory of our life, how we lived it, our values, what we believe. A part of ourselves lives on. A legacy can be something monumental for a whole society, like the Declaration of Independence, or something meaningful to a family, such as Great-grandma's recipe for chicken soup or banana bread, a city park named for a family member who was a prominent citizen, a flower garden originally planted by someone's father, or a passion for justice that shaped both a private and a public life such as Ken's. Our legacy is how we live on in our families and communities. How we live our lives is our gift to our world.

1. What experiences have you had with someone who was unable to accept dependence? How did you handle that and what did you learn?

2. How can you help someone keep some independence yet ease the sadness and disappointment of the losses?

3. Have you ever thought about what your legacy might include? How might you choose your work, volunteer commitments, political decisions, or conversations to reflect who you are and what you want people to know about you? How would you help someone else to think about his or her legacy?

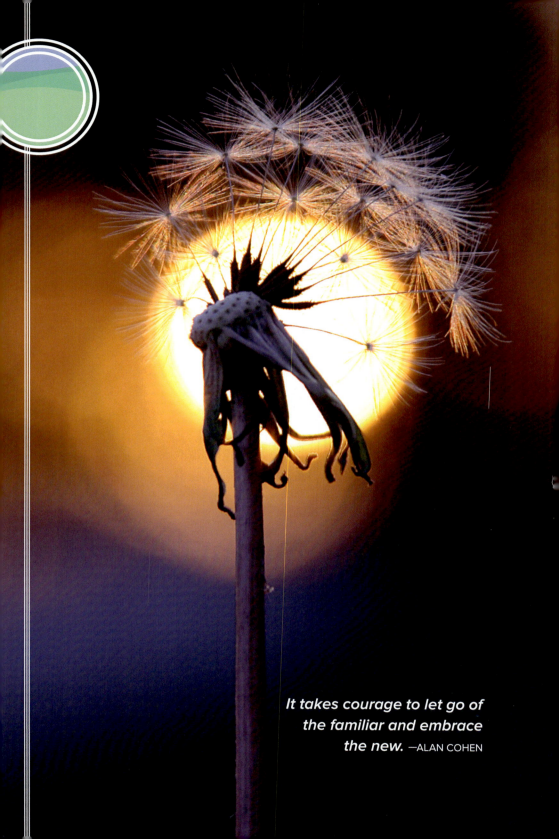

RUTH
LIFE IS FULL OF JOY

THE LARGE AUDITORIUM WAS FILLED WHEN THE DALAI LAMA visited our city a year ago. I immediately noticed Ruth standing a few feet away from where I was sitting. She had a broad smile and was personally greeted by whomever walked by. She was stunning, tall, and elegantly dressed. Then I noticed her arm. What I mean to say is I saw that her left arm ended just past her elbow. She didn't seem a bit self-conscious as she raised her right arm to emphasize what she was saying and her partial left arm came up too.

My first thought was that I'd really be interested in knowing her story. Someone who knew both of us walked by, and in the mutual greeting I was introduced to Ruth. I called her the following week, and she graciously accepted my invitation to share a conversation. Her tale was one of a very healthy woman who received a life-changing diagnosis. This is how Ruth began telling her story.

I'm sixty-two now. I was a fifty-four-year-old wife and mother, and soon to be a grandmother, and I was well and physically active. I did daily meditation and yoga, attended church regularly, and volunteered in my community. I read stories to four-year-olds in two different locations every week. That was a pretty normal life.

For seven weeks I was aware of a strange discomfort inside my left wrist. I went to my doctor and he did X-rays, an MRI, a complete examination, and a biopsy. After that examination my doctor sent me to an orthopedic surgeon, who simply said, "You have a soft tissue sarcoma that is very rare. It's cancer." The doctor showed me a mass four inches long inside my hand and up into my wrist. I had never heard of the disease before. With some hesitation, he told me that something like this keeps growing and eventually would metastasize in my lungs.

I have a gynecologist friend who helped me better understand the research. When I saw the specialist again, I was able to come with an intelligent list of questions that my friend had provided for me. One was, "What will happen as the mass in my left arm keeps growing?" He responded directly and honestly, "If you do nothing about this, it will kill you." Now I had to make a decision about whether to go ahead with the amputation. I thought about all the changes I'd have to deal with living with one arm. I'm an active person and work out at the gym at least five days a week. I'm often out in public socially and host events related to my husband's business, and I do volunteer work with young children. An enormous challenge would be that I'm left-handed. I knew I'd have to agree to the surgery to save my life. I cried all the way home. For three months before the surgery, I had chemotherapy to shrink the tumor. The bad news, and also the good news, about the chemo was that it didn't help shrink the tumor at all. That meant I wouldn't need further chemo after the surgery.

I had to deal with a physical adjustment, and also dramatic emotional and psychological changes. The physical adjustment was the hardest for me, but it gave me something to focus on. I was determined to be able to wash my face and comb my hair and put on my makeup. I made a list of what I needed to learn and worked with an occupational therapist. The first challenge I took on, because I had been left-handed, was to learn how to be right-handed as well as one-handed. I had to learn how to button my jeans, hook my bra, tie my shoes—all those things a person does without thinking about them, that I now couldn't do with one arm.

I knew immediately that, having half an arm, I couldn't hide something people view as a disability and a limitation. Maintaining a sense of humor was very important. It helped me with some of the long learning processes, and it kept people around me comfortably engaged with me while I was learning. Some ways I have to do things now are really pretty funny. For example, I learned to tie my shoes with my teeth by pulling my leg across my knee, bending my head down so I can reach the shoelace with my teeth. I've had to keep myself limber to accomplish those things, and I've discovered that being limber has other benefits too. I've had other experiences in my life where I've been in a fetal position on the floor in a puddle of tears from whatever crisis I was undergoing and not learned much from that response. Now I've learned things about myself that have helped me manage new challenges that come into my life.

I've always been a very persistent person, and I'm also a woman of faith. Sometimes faith can take care of my fears. I deeply believe that whatever happens, it's my job to do the best I can with it. It's all about acceptance of what is. Now I see that you don't always get to choose what happens to you, but you can choose your attitude toward any situation you're in. This was and still is the way that I've grown, living with one arm.

Now I am at a place in my life when I want to share with others what I've learned about myself through all this. And what I can say about being one-handed is that every day I'm confronted with a new challenge that requires two hands. I've learned to ask for help and accept it with a thank you and not expect impossible things from myself. I want people to understand, though, that I have my down moments, and they probably would too. I recall a time when the amputation was quite new, and I would wake up in the morning and think about going to exercise at the gym like I always did, and I'd think, "Who wants to see you there like this?" My best answer was, "You do!"

I began building a speaking career to encourage others to help themselves. My main message is that change is inevitable, but growth is intentional. Changes can be large or small. Whether you believe that things happen by accident or design, change can challenge your family or personal life, your employment or finances, your health or living conditions. You might have to deal with the death of a loved one. When such things happen, they most often represent loss of one kind or another, the loss of a dream or a goal, a loved one or a body part, a job or a position or a relationship. Whatever, life is full of personal loss. When you acknowledge the loss, then you have to grieve. I've now learned that grieving can be a process of discovery, not only of what was lost but also of what remains and of what is possible.

One thing I always mention is how important keeping a sense of humor has been. Keeping some lightness in my life is a big one for me. I have also learned that even if you do all the so-called right things—eat a balanced diet, do yoga and exercise regularly, volunteer in your community, help others, all those good things—you can still get cancer anyway!

I feel that people often want me to assure them that embracing what is will be relatively easy. They want to believe that it isn't so much work. But it is. You can stick your head in the sand and not deal with whatever changes or challenges come your way, but that isn't going to give you the opportunity to grow. When a person needs to adapt to a change, big or small, a conscious effort needs to be made to some new arrangement in your life. You need to be patient, to work on keeping a quiet mind and an open heart. You say quietly to yourself that you've made the adjustment, and then another day some other change comes into your life and you need to make a new adaptation. What I've learned is what I want to continue teaching in any way I can. A talk that I gave the other day was entitled "Growing through the Narrow Spots." That's what my disease and the amputation have helped me learn, and my mission now is to encourage others to grow though their narrow spots.

Out of this life-changing event in my life I've discovered a way to help others face the changes and challenges that come into their lives. I sincerely believe that I might be able to help and even inspire people who would listen and hear about unexpected, unplanned challenges in their lives. The purpose of telling my story in public or in private conversation is to let people know that we all have the resources to confront whatever faces us in our lives.

Thankfully, I'm now eight years out, so I'm pretty much sure I can call myself cancer-free. Now I deliver my message in a variety of public presentations, speeches, and workshops. I hope to encourage people to embrace their reality with a positive, life-affirming approach. This is more than my cancer story. I often repeat the phrase that change is inevitable but growth is intentional. It's about change and how you, I, everyone embraces one's own changes. I read a quote once that I often think about, because it captures the meaning of what I believe. It goes something like this: "I don't want to get to the end of my life and find that I lived just the length of it. I want to have lived both the width and the depth of it too."

I have great admiration for Ruth's career as an inspirational speaker. I've witnessed a couple of her presentations, and the audiences have been attentive and appreciative as she tells of her fears, her struggles, her determination, and her resulting victories. She offers her story to others as a gift, and she offers it with humor and sincerity. She donates the honoraria and fees she gathers to the cancer research fund at her local university medical school.

I see from Ruth's honesty about her relearning experience that it takes patience, courage, and commitment to accomplish what she has done. She's demonstrated the ability to put impatience aside, learned to give herself appreciation for small learnings, and continually reinforced her determination to reach her goal to live as normally as possible. I've also seen her stay for a long while following her public appearances to talk with attendees who are seeking personal encouragement and support.

Ruth's recent book, *Growing Through the Narrow Spots,* offers distilled wisdom and inspiration. Her monthly e-mails offer images of nature's beauty and simple words of wisdom. I carry Ruth's story with me through the narrow parts of my life and gain personal strength from her determination to persevere. I often share her story with others. One brief quote from her book says it all: "Don't just go through the narrow spots, grow through them."

1. What conversations have you had with persons who have dealt with amputations or drastic physical changes and challenges that require relearning how to use parts of their bodies? How have you been able to offer encouragement and hope to them?

2. How might you use Ruth's story and the stories of others who have succeeded at relearning and the recovery of their confidence and independence?

3. What have you learned from Ruth's story that has helped you personally or professionally? What have you gained from Ruth's story?

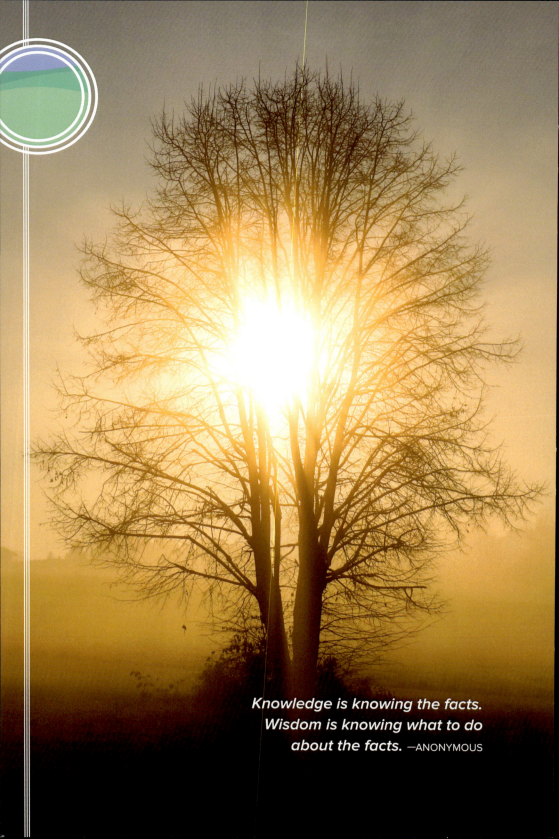

KATRINA
A GOOD LIFE

MEETING KATRINA, A HIGH-LEVEL UNIVERSITY ADMINISTRATOR, you would encounter a lively, attractive, well-dressed woman soon approaching fifty. If you were one of the school's graduate students or faculty members, you'd probably know some of her personal story. I asked her to share the details of her many physical challenges. Some health conditions are lifetime battles. We each have our own challenges, and we never know whose story might offer us motivation and inspiration to handle our own. This is a story of endurance and determination. Meet Katrina. I hope her story will be as meaningful to you as it was to me.

I was nineteen when I got out of bed one morning and couldn't feel my legs. I fell to the floor, and I could hardly get up. That was the beginning of a long journey that I'm still on. This was in the early 1980s, and it took considerable time back then to get a confirmed diagnosis of multiple sclerosis. During the year after I fell, the doctors tested for everything else as I became increasingly disabled. I was bedridden, in a wheelchair, and constantly having to make adjustments because of my illness.

I read every book I could find about people who dealt with disabilities in their lives. Helen Keller was an inspiration to me in a very dark moment. In spite of all the challenges she faced, she went to college, and I needed that kind of encouragement. I learned something else from her. She accepted help when it was offered. Although asking for help was hard for me, it's an ongoing need for me, and I've learned to do that too. I've discovered that allowing people to help me is a kindness, because most people sincerely want to do something. I'll always remember the people who have been there for me.

I have had so many teachers who helped me, along with wonderful caregivers who believed in me. I knew I had to immerse myself in a positive environment, so if a caregiver or an acquaintance was negative, I quickly let the person go. I responded to caregivers who believed in me. I couldn't focus on my goals if someone who was assigned to care for me came in and said something like, "Too bad you'll never walk again" or "It's sad you'll never see the Grand Canyon." That person wasn't invited back. I learned through all this to be stronger.

I knew what my priorities were, and I kept them in focus. After high school some of my friends went off to college. I felt abandoned by many, but one good friend stuck with me. I guess the others just didn't know how to handle my situation. That friend would talk with me about my goals, and she'd rub my feet and say things that made me laugh. Small acts of kindness can have a big impact.

I've learned to live in my head, because I couldn't rely on my body. I wanted to continue to learn, and I chose to go to a small liberal arts college for women, although I couldn't easily attend classes regularly. My teachers were supportive. They did something very special for me by sending all the books for my courses to a group that made audio recordings for the blind. I had double vision at the time and couldn't read, but by listening to my books on tape, I could keep up. My teachers allowed me to do my exams orally. I missed out on the experience of sharing in classroom interaction, but some students who came to visit me at home were very helpful. We had conversations that were important to me. I managed to graduate from college, and by that time my health was a bit better, so I went on to graduate school. I saw that my only avenue for success was education. I wanted to teach, and I didn't need my body for that, just my mind.

When I was in my twenties, I was completely overlooked by the world of twenty-year-old women who were getting married and having babies. I saw very quickly that people make assumptions about anyone they think of as "not normal." Whatever the social norms are, they assume you aren't able to participate. They kept me on the outside. Being disabled when you're twenty is like suddenly turning eighty. I found that I rapidly became invisible or disregarded by others, particularly when I was in a wheelchair. If I was in a department store, restaurant, or airport, I became like an infant to people who wouldn't talk to me but would talk to my caregiver. They'd say things like, "Does she want anything?" and I'd answer, "You can address me." It was a common experience then, and regrettably, it still is.

I seemed to get stronger as time went on, and eventually, at age twenty-seven, I became ambulatory. That was over twenty years ago. During that time I've had intermittent problems and have had to use crutches or a walker and occasionally a wheelchair. I now know the reason I gradually got better. They've discovered that MS is of two types. There's a chronic progressive form and a relapsing remitting one, which is what I have. It's still progressive and chronic, but it's developing much more slowly, and I go through long periods of remission. I've received a lot of cortisone and steroids and a good deal of physical therapy over the years. It's not in my nature to give up, and I've been determined to live as normally as possible in spite of the times when I've experienced sadness, frustration, and anger about my illness. My life lesson is that I've learned to turn those feelings into determination.

I believe that as we get older we learn to integrate both our good and our bad experiences and to see benefits from both. Sometimes I'm with someone who's now in her midforties, and she's talking about her youth. I'm sitting there thinking, "I never had a youth." I went from adolescence to feeling like I was ancient! I'm working on recovering my youth. Now in my forties, I've captured a liveliness and lightness that I certainly didn't have when I was twenty. I prefer to be with older people, because my illness catapulted me through the life cycle. In a strange and beautiful way, sometimes I feel I have that wisdom of an older person. Younger persons are still working out their issues and spending time with stuff that really doesn't matter to me or how I live my life.

People often ask me if religious beliefs are a support for me. I actually call myself an atheist. I've come to the position that there is no god in the Judeo-Christian sense, but I do believe there's a god in all of us. I belong to a group that supports humanistic values. The positive connections we make with each other are, to me, godlike. It's a very spiritual thing. I don't usually talk about this, because people have their own beliefs. I don't want to hurt people in my own family who have other religious beliefs and practices, and I don't want to argue about it. I do believe in human beings and our capacity for love, kindness, and generosity. I believe, too, in our own goodness and our ability to work for justice.

I have very busy days with my work. It helps me feel validated and valued. I know that I always want to be the strongest person in the room. I see myself behaving this way because of being disabled. I often do things that are really stupid; for example, I have never taken a sick day. I struggle with that sometimes, knowing I shouldn't go to work, but it's so important to me that I go. I don't want anyone ever to say that I took sick leave because I couldn't do the job. Still, I know if I access my inner wisdom more regularly, I'll let myself be a human being. I want to be able to take a day off when I have a fever or a cold or just plain feel sick, in consideration for others and my own needs. I'm working on learning to accept doing that.

I've done a good deal of meditation and contemplation and a lot of visualization and guided imagery, which have helped me enormously. This past year I had to have major surgery because of tumors in my spine, and I used those tools that I had developed in my twenties to help my recovery. They all kicked back in, and I constantly focused on being well. I used homeopathic medications, I got out of the hospital three days early, and I had very little scarring. I healed so well because I had all those skills already, and I just needed them to kick back in. Those support skills I developed and used in earlier difficult years continue to be accessible to me every day.

Life is incredibly fragile. Something can happen to anyone at any time. I've truly learned to appreciate every moment. I know how important it is to be in the present. I never know when I'm going to wake up and have double vision or have to go back in a wheelchair or whatever. There are times when I still get angry about my illness, and then I remind myself that I have to live in the here and now. I'm in a plateau with my MS at the moment. I don't look ahead. I just live every day.

I make an effort to bring what I've learned into where I am

right now. We can share our experiences, our learning, and our wisdom, and we can stay open to learn from others. We're all on different paths. One lesson I learned from being cared for is the value of listening to people. So many times I've listened to whoever was visiting just talk. I feel that I've had some very beautiful and meaningful friendships develop from people's trust, and through all this, I've learned a lot about being cared for from those who have visited me often and truly acknowledged me. I got through those early years with the help of others and learned that it takes a village, as the expression goes. I think of an old Ojibwa saying that translated means, "I see you." It's truly a gift to have people in my life who have tried to see the me inside.

> **A strong positive mental attitude will create more miracles than any wonder drug.** —PATRICIA NEAL

Learning to take care of ourselves is a challenge for many of us. Obstacles come into each of our lives, and we need to remember that taking care of ourselves is necessary to do our best work and serve others well. We don't always know what details from someone's personal story can give us answers, inspiration, or an insight that can change our own response to some personal challenge. Katrina's lifelong determination continues to strengthen and support her, whatever comes along in her life. It can inspire us too. I met a former student from the graduate program of the university where Katrina teaches, and she told me how knowing some of the challenges Katrina had faced and seeing how she dealt with her illness and built her life had given her the courage and determination to go back to her own studies after a necessary amputation.

As we concluded our conversation, Katrina offered a closing thought: "The secret is that if we are kind to ourselves and to others, we can help our world begin to shift in a more hopeful way." I am truly grateful to Katrina for the gift of her determination to serve herself so she can serve others.

1. Have you had any experience with persons who have been dealing with a difficult condition or limitation for their whole lifetime? If so, have they dealt with setbacks? How have you best served and supported them?

2. What insights about aging can you gain from Katrina's comment that her opinions and attitudes are more similar to an older person's than to those of someone her own age?

3. What is the most powerful message for you in Katrina's story? How can you help others in your life benefit from her attitude and perseverance?

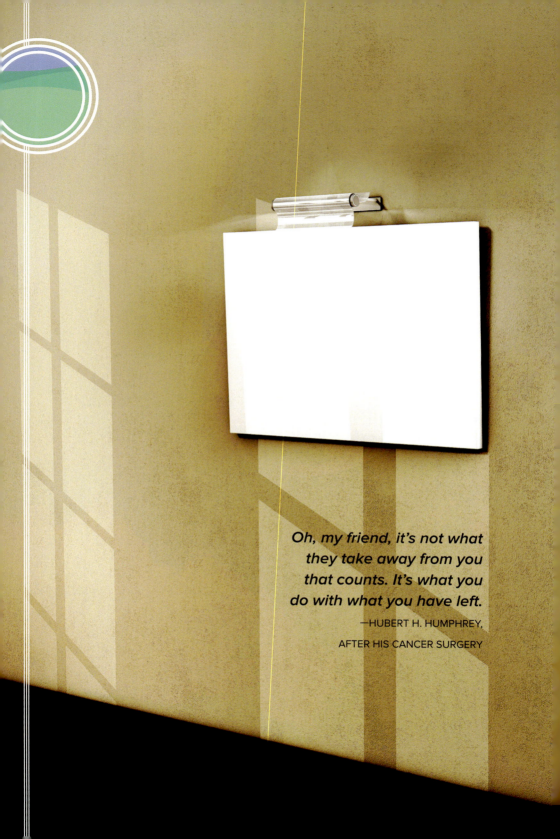

> Oh, my friend, it's not what they take away from you that counts. It's what you do with what you have left.
> —HUBERT H. HUMPHREY, AFTER HIS CANCER SURGERY

GARY
A LIFE OF HELPING OTHERS

GARY WAS ONE OF THE FOUNDERS OF SAGE-ING, NOW SAGE-ING International, an organization founded in 2004 based on the writings and philosophy of the late Rabbi Zalman Schachter-Shalomi and his book *From Age-ing to Sage-ing*. Sage-ing isn't a religious practice; it's a way of living the second half of our lives that is joyful, fulfilling, and useful. The philosophy and practice of sage-ing involves both personal and spiritual growth based on the belief that aging offers unexplored opportunities for discovering new insights, deepening spirituality, and developing positive perspectives for living a meaningful later life.

Gary's life and work is now dedicated to helping elders honor the values of lifelong learning, service, community, respect, integrity, engaged leadership, and compassion, and to reclaim their role as leaders in our society. In our conversation he told me what his life had once been, how he was enjoying his so-called retirement, and how a surgeon's slip of the knife changed everything.

I'll begin telling my story about when I was a research scientist and a technician at a national laboratory. I retired from that profession when my company downsized, because I was interested in doing many other things. I was only fifty-six at that time. I was a potter, and I loved that, so I took it on full time when I left my job. I showed my work in art galleries and other venues for many years.

Another of my activities was working as a hospice volunteer. My parents were getting older, and I wanted to get more familiar with death, a subject I hadn't given much thought to in my earlier years. This led to my developing a deeper personal perspective about my spiritual side and becoming involved in the beginning of the Sage-ing organization. However, my body wasn't as healthy as my spirit. I developed spine problems that became extremely limiting, and I needed a cervical spine fusion to solve some problems in my neck. The surgery corrected the neck problems, but during the operation the surgeon had accidentally cut a nerve that controls one half of my vocal cords. Very soon I realized I couldn't talk at all. The doctor said recovery might take a few months, but after a time there was no improvement in my voice. At that point my doctor said that if I hadn't recovered my ability to talk normally in a year, I would probably never get my voice back.

I was fortunate, because my voice did begin to come back slowly. The cut nerve hasn't ever repaired itself, and my voice hasn't returned to what it had been. Playing guitar and singing had become an important part of my life, but I lost both volume and clarity and no longer have any vocal range. When I could speak again I was self-conscious about my quiet, gravelly voice and wondered if I really could be understood. I tried speaking in small groups and learned that people got used to my voice. They asked me to repeat what they couldn't understand and it wasn't a big issue for me or them.

I tried to do whatever I could with doctors and speech therapists, hoping to make my voice better. Those efforts helped, although I can't be heard in a noisy restaurant, for example, or even in a room with others talking. But I love to be with people and can share conversation successfully in a very quiet place or in a quiet, one-to-one conversation. But that's the best I can do. I've come to accept that my voice will never again be strong. I don't think so much about it anymore.

During the time of my partial recovery, my wife reminded me many times that learning to accept my new limitation was in reality a gift. It actually put me in touch with the fragility of us all. I really believe that the loss of my voice and my ability to engage in other activities have really taught me something important about myself. I often quote the violinist Itzhak Perlman, who has lived since the age of forty without the use of his legs as a result of polio. He has many times said, "I'm glad to have what I have left and to make the most of my life with that." This is what I sincerely believe, and I hope that is now the message of my teaching.

It certainly has also helped me to have a supportive wife throughout this time. Charlotte has continued to be a cheerleader for me and is often a co-teacher with me. She always makes me smile when she says I'm a kinder person these days. Losing my voice was a humbling experience and probably has made me more sensitive to other persons and their disabilities.

The other thing that's probably been in my favor is that I seem to have a number of talents, so the loss of this one ability was not as devastating to me as it might otherwise have been.

I think it has to do with my understanding that we all are likely to lose some of our capabilities as we grow older, and this early loss made it easier for me to accept those realities. I live with the philosophy that we are best served by accepting some of the inevitable "slings and arrows of outrageous fortune" that we encounter. That attitude works pretty well for me.

I was seventy-one on my last birthday and slowly realizing that my disability and my aging might be the seeds of a new and meaningful activity. I spent a good deal of time wondering whether I could be effective working as a teacher and group leader. It took me quite a while before I was able to make that decision. I'm now working with people interested in their own aging, and dealing with challenging situations they are facing. Doing that work with others became a passion for me and very quickly became greater than my concerns about my voice. I no longer can do public speeches or radio broadcasts, but I can teach small classes. I've helped many people with end-of-life issues and a variety of second-half-of-life concerns.

This change in my life has taught me that things can change in a hurry and that we don't often have control over those changes. We all have within us the capacity for resilience, and we can live with losses and still have a good life. Life is all about choices. Even when losses are great or choices are difficult, looking at the good part of our lives is necessary to sustain us. We can learn about ourselves and grow from facing adversity. I believe that, and I teach that. When I've taught my small groups, I've heard over and over again about things happening that we don't plan and we don't want. The secret is to choose to do what you can with whatever situation or limitation you're facing. We can experience more joyful moments with that perspective than if we are always looking at the problems. That's the attitude I attempt to teach and how I try to live. People in my classes light up when they see some of the possibilities and opportunities they never realized before.

I've adjusted to the reality of my situation, and I can honestly say, "Here I am, and I'm happy with who I am." I've made the choice to go on with my life as normally as I can with what I have left. People are faced with their own challenges and choices and have to adjust to what they have to deal with. So many people who have been in my classes have had close encounters with death, either themselves or with a loved one. Almost without exception I can say the learning from such experiences has resulted in personal growth. There's an honest acceptance that life is fragile, that we don't know everything about our future and can't control everything. Like those I teach, I can come through losses and gain profound insights along with a new and deep appreciation of daily life.

I look at my glass half full, not half empty. That attitude is important in what I teach. Aging well, aging consciously, requires a person to try to sustain that attitude no matter what his or her reality is. I realized that I had a choice of focusing on and staying with the pain of my lost voice or moving on and accepting my limitation. For the most part I've come to peace with the loss. I quoted Itzhak Perlman earlier in our conversation; another story he often tells is about a time when a violin string broke during a concert performance and he continued to play using the remaining strings. At the end of the performance he said, "Sometimes you just have to do the best you can with what you have left." That's a good metaphor for the aging journey. That's how I now feel about the loss of my voice. I remember when I felt I would have to give up teaching, but I still wanted to be with others who might learn from me, so I soldiered on.

I lost my voice, but I didn't lose my personhood. I'm one of the lucky ones. I'm at a stage of life when I can really explore being myself. I want to continue growing and teaching. My paid career is over, my children are grown, my life goes on, and I keep learning. I would not be teaching positive aging if I didn't truly believe it is possible. My goal is to make deeper connections with friends and family, develop new passions, and give back through service to others. I truly believe that these are my best years. In reality, this has become the most satisfying time of my life.

> **Life is change. Growth is optional. Choose wisely.** —KAREN KAISER CLARK

In our conversation, Gary said, "I've made the choice to go on with my life as normally as I can with what I have left," a life with an unexpected physical limitation. Decisions of such gravity often require a long process of reconciliation and integration into one's reality. Sometimes the steps to recovery from and learning how to live with a loss—whether the death of a loved one or friend, loss of a body part or a lifelong career, or changes to one's health and body that might come with the aging process—are very slow. When a way of living is no longer a choice, reading or hearing a story of someone who has embraced such a challenge and found new depth and meaning in his or her life can open a door to a new way of thinking.

An accident, a diagnosis of an illness, or any number of unexpected events can change our lives. I've so often heard the expression, "Life is what happens while we're making other plans." We never know when we might be the person requiring care. The cause might be a broken leg; it could be a diagnosis of an incurable disease. It also could be a loss of strength, versatility, or other changes and limitations that might come with an aging body. Both temporary and permanent disabilities can present us with an opportunity to look at our lives from a different perspective.

The mission of Sage-ing International is to change society's understanding of aging. We don't have to settle for simply becoming old; we can age consciously and learn what the elder years can offer. Many other national organizations and local groups, churches, and other services now host gatherings of persons in midlife and beyond to discuss these things. Some offer personal growth programs and assistance with whatever losses, illnesses, or diminishments are confronting people. They all promote the idea that we can each acquire insights and wisdom that offer a future of a deep and meaningful life.

1. Have you or someone close to you experienced changes in health or life circumstances that require major shifts in behavior, schedules, plans, and goals? What have you learned about accepting help and some measure of dependency? What stories might you share about your helping others with such challenges?

2. What differences and similarities do you see between (a) a younger person dealing with an amputation, a debilitating disease, or a life-changing injury or changes in health and (b) a diagnosis of an incurable disease at a later stage of life?

3. What have you learned from your work with others or in your personal life about the ways acceptance of negative or unexpected changes can open the door to a deeper and fuller life?

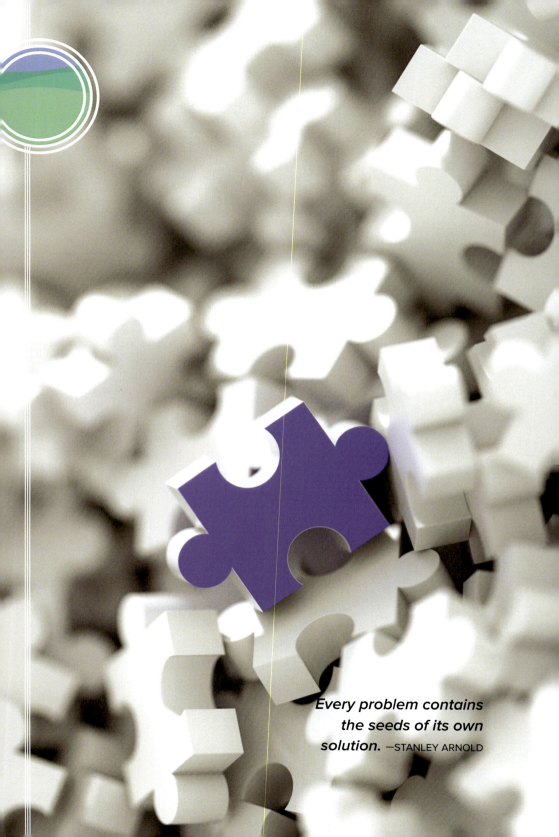

BILL
HELPING OTHERS SEEK A GOOD LIFE

I WAS ATTENDING A CONFERENCE WHEN A LARGE, FRIENDLY DOG came up to me and stood by my side. A short, smiling man followed and introduced me to his guide dog, Farley. As we were both waiting in line for a table at lunch, we decided to eat together. Bill's story of inner strength, persistence, determination, and adaptation turned out for me to be the best thing on the lunch menu.

I'm sixty-three years old now. I've survived a heart attack, massive blood clots, and open-heart surgery. I've also accommodated a life of visual disability. I'm considered legally blind, but I do have some very limited vision. My glasses are like thick bottles. I've learned how to live with barriers, to adapt, as they say, to live outside the box. But most important, I still have my passion for life.

I've always been treated differently and still am. Even today, here at lunch, a man came over to me and asked, "Why do you have a seeing eye dog when you obviously can see?" The truth is I really have extremely limited vision. I'm sitting right next to you, but I can't see the features of your face. I've learned my way around this particular facility, so my dog, Farley, follows me around instead of him leading me. When I leave this room and when I leave this building, I'll rely totally on him. I really need him to guide me. He's sees the doors, the steps, the curbs, and the traffic.

My mother was always my champion. She told me I could do anything I wanted to, and I believed her. When I was growing up, visually impaired people were treated as defective. When I was in sixth grade the teacher said that she couldn't deal with a blind child in her class, so I was put in a school for blind children for much of my early education. After we moved into a different home, I was enrolled in a different junior high school. It was a regular public school, and I was given large-print books.

It seems like I always had to fight for what I needed so I could keep on with my learning. Society was very cruel to people with disabilities when I was growing up in the 1950s and '60s. After high school, I chose to go to a Christian college, and the people there were very protective of me. My first degree was in religion, and I always felt that the church was a safe haven. I went back to school again when I was in my midfifties. I worked hard to memorize the material I needed to know for the entrance exams. I got a master's degree in public administration and found a good position dealing with programs for the aging, public policy, and other related areas. I saw advancement in the field of aging was available to me, so I made a plan to go back to school once again and work toward a PhD.

Things were interrupted for me when I had a massive heart attack during the fourth year I was back at the university. I guess my determination got me through the many months of recovery. I prayed a good deal; God and I have a good relationship. I believe I had a near-death experience when I had the heart attack, and I remember hearing my dead mother's voice saying, "It's not your time to come here yet." I always felt that I survived because I have a purpose in life. That has been my personal philosophy.

When I had almost completed my doctorate program, I changed my adviser, and the new person asked what technology I was using. I told her I didn't have anything but my thick reading glasses. I used a computer but set the print size at sixteen or eighteen. She told me about new screen-reading programs. They identify and interpret what's on the screen and then present it to me in speech. I followed up on that immediately and had them installed on my regular computer and my laptop. My computer now has a program that reads books to me, and I also have a very large screen and can make the print as large as seventy-eight points.

I teach at California State University in public health and also social work and gerontology. That's the work I've been doing and what I plan to continue doing. My teaching involves educating people about aging and caregiving. All my classes focus on continuing to live with purpose and passion. As for me personally, there are practical reasons for me to continue to be employed, besides the fact that I love my work. As long as I'm working, I have good medical coverage. The medications I take are very expensive. I'd never be able to afford what I need, and I'm thankful that my policy now covers it all.

I, like many older people, often have to deal with limitations. People with obvious limitations are often not thought of as part of an active society. I have all my students interview elders in a variety of situations and get to know them. I want my students to learn to be the voice of the disability or limitation another person is living with. I also have them observe closely how the world out there reflects elders in greeting cards, advertising, newspaper articles, and other media. An underlying ageism controls our society. I want my students to see this reality and the value of each individual. I want them to do what they can to combat such attitudes in the work they'll do some day. We need people in the field who have not only a passion for the work, but also compassion and honest understanding for elders as people.

I feel I have a mission in my work, and I've recently taken on a new project. I'm interviewing elders who are now in an assisted living residence. Everyone I've talked with has commented on the loneliness. It's a sad reflection on our society that we so often aren't in close touch with aged parents or other older people who live in relative isolation. I've found that so many of these people have great stories. They're repositories of history, and they're happy to share their memories and knowledge with me.

Those who have physical limitations have told me how they acquired their disability and how they're surviving. That has led to conversation about how the aides and other helpers in these residences often treat those who can't walk or who spend all day in a wheelchair. Many of the people I've had conversations with have survived a heart attack, cancer, or some other disabling illness, and often I hear of times when they're no longer treated like a functioning person. The people who help them in the home tend to focus totally on the illness, the disability, and the person's limitation. It's really sad to me that all too often they ignore the person inside the broken body.

I want to teach my colleagues, doctors, and those involved with both the teaching and the care of elders to acknowledge them as whole persons, even if their bodies are no longer whole. We have to start changing the system. I've talked about this with my cardiologist, internist, and urologist. They agree that the pressures of their profession don't allow the time to get to know the "inside" of a person. Their focus is almost totally on the physical problems. That's also true for so many others who work in senior care residences.

Whatever I can do to change things, to open up the medical world to these realities, to teach my students, to keep learning with them, I'll continue doing it. The advice I give is that all of us have to become our own advocate. We need to think about how we can overcome barriers or limitations to whatever disability or disease we're dealing with. We all have a purpose for being here, and we each need to do what we can to make our lives meaningful. We're not all writers, teachers, cooks, inventors, actors, poets, or whatever. We don't all have families around to spend time with us. We need to be encouraged to adapt to whatever challenges face us throughout our lives, to find what is meaningful and pleasurable to us, what will give us a satisfying day. I want to help people do that for themselves.

I've got a purpose, a mission, something that I care about with a passion. I want to help others continue to grow, to learn, to be seen as part of the world, no matter what limitations come with their circumstances and stage of life. That's now the meaning and purpose in my life.

I don't follow precedent, I establish it. —FANNY ELLEN HOTZMAN

Any comments I might offer would add little to Bill's story, but I'm eager to support his passion. I strongly agree with Bill's observation that many people often ignore the person inside an old or in some way disabled body. His teachings are aimed at young people to help them see and know the person despite his or her physical challenges. In our culture many persons are fearful or lack sensitivity or understanding about how to connect with such people. Our society has too long isolated people from normal, everyday interactions. I join Bill in striving to change those prejudiced perceptions that dominate attitudes and actions today.

Bill's words and his efforts offer others a more honest and rich image of the elderly and disabled. Our society desperately needs a more inclusive attitude about disabled, physically limited, or frail elderly. I hope that those reading this book will, like me, feel grateful to Bill for bringing such prejudicial responses to our awareness and, like me, check out their immediate, unconscious negative reactions to encounters with elderly and disabled persons.

1. **Have you had any experience of helping a person with limited vision? How have you (or would you) offer assistance? What words might you avoid? What about the tone of your voice? What do your words and how you say them communicate about your attitude toward the person's dependency?**

2. **What are your observations about ageism in our society? What incidents have you witnessed with disfigured, obviously disabled, or elderly persons that reveal unspoken fears and prejudice? What reservations do you have about encountering people with limitations of any kind?**

3. **What stories might you share that illustrate such prejudiced and fearful behavior, or your learning or unlearning such behaviors?**

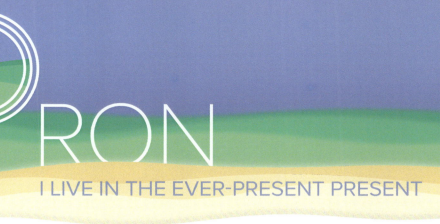

RON
I LIVE IN THE EVER-PRESENT PRESENT

There is just one path for each of us—our own. —EURIPIDES

ONCE UPON A TIME RON HELD AN EXECUTIVE POSITION AT A bank in the city where he, his wife, and two sons lived. I met Ron, who now is in his eighties, in our local YMCA swimming pool. In the early morning on weekdays, a few of us do our own version of the water aerobics instructor's movements in the pool. For many years Ron has had severe arthritis. His body is bent, and he walks stooped over with slow small steps. The range of his movement out of the water is severely limited. He can't walk very far with any comfort, but he relishes his ability to move freely in the pool, where he can ignore his physical limitations.

His most recent regular annual physical resulted in a diagnosis of colon cancer. Following this diagnosis was surgery and many months of recovery. One day he appeared at the pool with a smile on his face. We again were able to enjoy many good conversations.

Many months later, Ron's wife was in ill health. He and their grown sons became her caregivers. That ended our morning swim, and our friendship turned into an e-mail correspondence. One day we decided that two sentences in an e-mail didn't always satisfy, so I set up a time for a conversation with Ron at his home. I was confident that he would have some words of encouragement and wisdom for anyone facing a diagnosis that forced unexpected changes in his or her regular routine. He met me at the door and made some remark about how lucky we were to recognize each other in our clothes instead of our bathing suits. Ron's smile and sense of humor were alive and well. We went into his comfortable living room, he sat in his favorite chair, and our conversation began with the story of the annual physical checkup where it was discovered that he had colon cancer.

I casually mentioned to my doctor that I had noticed a little blood in my stool recently. A colonoscopy was scheduled, and my doctor told me almost immediately that I had problems. He made an appointment for me to see a surgeon that very day. One of my sons is a nurse, and I took him with me to that appointment so I could have someone there to explain what I might not understand.

The colonoscopy revealed a mass, actually two of them. One was in the upper portion of my colon and another in the lower region. The doctor explained the surgery was extensive, and that I would have to wear an appliance, a bag to accommodate my elimination process for the rest of my life. I asked what would be the consequences if I didn't do the surgery. Dying from colon cancer isn't pleasant, he told me, and he strongly recommended I schedule the surgery.

I've heard many stories these past years from friends and acquaintances about cancer surgeries that resulted in unpleasant chemo treatments and difficult days in their remaining years. I didn't want to live my last days that way. I may have made the decision to forego the surgery, but my son said, "Dad, I think you should follow the doctor's advice and go through the surgery." There I was with a doctor whose profession is to treat and prolong life, and a son who doesn't want to lose his dad. As my general attitude is one of optimism, the surgery was scheduled. I was really at peace with the decision once it was made, and I am now. I decided to go along with the process, and my attitude was total acceptance. I don't know if that's usual, but that's how I am. Following the surgery I was told that it was totally successful. Then I had to adjust to the necessary changes. That was two years ago, when I had just turned eighty.

With the doctor's permission and encouragement, I was told that after I healed from the surgery I could return to my regular water exercise. The day I appeared at the pool I described to some of my regular colleagues the elimination bag that had become a permanent necessity. For several months after my surgery, I was able to join the morning swim. My adjustment to using what I call the bag took some time. My wife, Sylvia, has been my helper through it all. She's been supportive and encouraging, and that has been important to me both physically and emotionally. She's always there to help me replace the bag and clean up, and she's very patient. I can't give her any help, because the bag is in a location where I can't even see it.

I do feel limited by wearing the device. I'm apprehensive about going out to dinner at a restaurant or at someone's house. I have no way of predicting when the bag will fill up. My elimination pattern is out of my control. I'm sensitive to smells, and sometimes I hear gurgles and other noises when elimination happens. We do sometimes go out, and I enjoy that, but it's always in the back of my mind that the bag could fill. I'm always thinking about it when we're away from the house, but I do have much of my regular social life back now. At this time in my life I have everything I need. We have a comfortable home, I have a loving wife and grown children. In spite of the cancer, there's so much I'm thankful for in the precious present. That's the reality for me: right now. All I have, all every one of us really has, is this moment. For me, that's the key, the present.

For me, I'd say my attitude is religious based. I'm not a scholar of the Bible, but certain phrases have meant a good deal to me, and my basic belief is that there's a God. I can't imagine how this creation, this world of ours, could have come about without some power. And then there are human beings with eyes that see and ears that hear and hearts that function and cells that multiply. It's beyond my human mind. My faith makes me content with my life as it is.

There are things I can control and other things I can't. I learned this life lesson a long time ago. I've learned to keep a positive attitude about things I can control. Right now I'm at peace with what I have and how I'm living. I think each person is here for a purpose. I think I'm given this extra time for a purpose. I don't know what it actually could be, but I trust that thought.

I was exposed to the reality of the life cycle at a young age. I learned about death when my father bought me a rifle when I was about ten years old. My dad took me out into the grove and told me to always remember that when I shot a bird or anything living, it would be dead. I knew from an early age that when a living being was dead, there was no way to bring that life back. From that time on I realized life was something very, very precious. That knowledge is with me, and I know it deeply at this time of my life. My living each day is a gift, and I treasure it and live it consciously.

My days pass so quickly, and they're filled with things I never paid much attention to in the old days. But now I spend my morning dressing, shaving, brushing my teeth, taking my blood sugar and other medications, having breakfast, and reading the paper. I have four or five different doctors, and I need to keep track of my appointments before I get too involved with my day. I've found that when I have a day off from those commitments, looking back on my life has become my most enjoyable part of my todays. What a gift remembering is. I think about my childhood, school, marriage, children, jobs, work, friends, and the many people who have been and are now part of my life. I'm thankful for all my yesterdays, and that makes the todays so precious.

I remember reading a very small book quite a long time ago called *The Precious Present*. It was published more than thirty years ago, and it may have been on my shelf since. I've reread it three or more times during this past week. It has touched a deep belief in me about the importance of how I live at this time of my life. I'd like to tell some of the story to you.

Ron asked me to reach for the book on a nearby table. He explained that it told the tale of a boy growing through his childhood into young adulthood and then into middle age. The boy kept visiting an old man and always found him willing to talk about the gift of the precious present, and the boy remained open to listening.

He proceeded to tell me some of the story from the slim book he held tight in his hands.

Once there was a little boy who listened to an old man, and thus he began to learn about the precious present. The old man told the young boy, "It's a present, because it's a gift. And anyone who receives it is happy forever." As the young man went through his life, he kept searching for the precious present the old man had told him about. At times the young man thought he had it figured out and would go back to visit the old man again, only for the old man to say, "No, that's not it," and the young man would continue trying to find this precious gift. One day the old man died. The now middle-aged man had grown tired of looking so he stopped searching. It was then that he finally realized what the precious present was. It wasn't the past. It wasn't the future. It was the present. It was today. And the middle-aged man found his happiness.

As Ron's telling of the story was coming to a conclusion, I knew, as anyone listening or reading the story would know, that it had become important to the now old man to pass along the gift of the precious present and to teach his insights and life lessons to a young child. There were tears in Ron's eyes. He was quiet for a bit, and then he spoke.

I've now come to understand that when I'm totally in the present, in spite of what's going on in my personal world, my health or lack of it, or whatever, that I'm perfectly content to be where I am. I've learned from this simple story that the richness of the present comes from within. It isn't something someone gives to you. It's something you give to yourself. I think I always knew this, but I see now how vital it is to understand this life lesson in a deeper and more personal way. The precious present is just that: the present, not the past, not the future, but the precious present. That moment can evaporate. It's a process that a person has to do over and over again to unlearn those old habits of looking to the past or the future. A person has to be in the present to know the preciousness of that moment.

This little book speaks to me. For me it's the whole secret of how to live. Life isn't always easy or pleasant, but there's simplicity in this point of view if a person can hold on to it. Finding a way to stay in the here and now is my way of deliberately embracing the present. At this time of my life, the present is where my contentment resides.

> ***Decide to enjoy life to the fullest no matter what. Remember that each day is a good one just because you are alive.*** —ANONYMOUS

During Ron's telling of *The Precious Present,* I thought about what he had said to me earlier in our conversation: "I think I'm given this extra time for a purpose. I don't know what it actually could be, but I trust that thought." Possibly awakening others to the precious present is his current purpose and his precious gift. He shared the story and the wise words and insights it contains, and gave me the opportunity to pass on his precious gift.

I also continue to believe in the truth of a quote by the poet Muriel Rukeyser that I read many years ago. "The world isn't made of atoms, it's made of stories," she wrote. I sincerely believe that hearing a story opens to us the possibility of learning and growing. We laugh, cry, empathize, and we have the potential of learning something about ourselves in the often-changing circumstances of our own lives.

Reading or hearing a personal and poignant tale may offer us an unexpected source of comfort and inspiration. Wisdom and insight can come from someone we don't know and may never meet. Such is the power of story. With this thought, and with thanks to my friend Ron, I pass along the challenge and the gift he gave me of being present in the precious present. This is a gift to me, and I hope to the reader too.

1. When has a story you've heard or lived changed your opinion, actions, or work, or led you to make some dramatic change in your own life?

2. How has Ron's story influenced your work, your friendships and family relations, or possibly your caregiving responsibilities?

3. Why is it so difficult for many of us to stay in the present? How might we benefit if we could do that?

AFTERWORD

FOR MORE THAN FORTY YEARS I HAVE BEEN COLLECTING STORIES and giving those voices that have often been neglected a venue to be heard. Caregivers are conscientiously concerned with the physical needs of those in care. This is often the essence of the conversation between the caregiver and the one in care. I understand that those practical concerns, and also the overwhelming schedule of a caregiver, are of vital importance.

Some of what I have written and suggested may sound repetitious when I so often stress the need to go beyond addressing only physical needs in order to also provide friendly, informal, and humorous content in the exchange between the caregiver and the one in care. If we take the labels away, these are just two people in conversation. My hope is that more often, their dialogue might reflect the mutuality and reciprocity the word *exchange* implies.

ABOUT THE AUTHOR

Connie Goldman is an award-winning radio producer and reporter. Beginning her broadcast career with Minnesota Public Radio, she later worked for several years on the staff of National Public Radio in Washington D.C. For over the 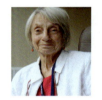 past 30 years her public radio programs, books, and speaking have been exclusively concerned with the changes and challenges of aging. Grounded in the art of personal stories collected from hundreds of interviews, Connie's presentations are designed to inform, empower, and inspire. Her message on public radio, in print and in person is clear—make any time of life an opportunity for new learning, exploring creative pursuits, self-discovery, spiritual deepening, and continued growth.